Fasting

The Ultimate Guide to Intermittent, Alternate-Day, and Extended Water Fasting and How to Activate Autophagy for Weight Loss and Anti-Aging

Contents

Part 1: Water Fasting

Unlock the Secrets of Weight Loss, Anti-Aging, Autophagy, and Ketosis with Intermittent, Alternate-Day, and Extended Fasting

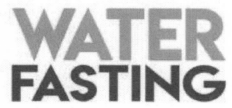

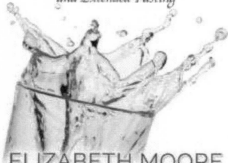

Introduction

You've heard a lot about water fasting nowadays. It seems like the latest weight loss fad that has caught on in a big way. Let me tell you straight up here—it is here to stay because it has tons of benefits if done correctly. There are plenty of misconceptions and myths regarding water fasting that we will burst along the way. However, it is here to stay, which is why you must know its benefits and how to use it correctly. Let us first understand the concept of water fasting.

What is water fasting all about?

Fasting is a form of restricting intake of food, which has been practiced since ancient times for several purposes including religion. Water fasting is a kind of fasting that limits a person from eating everything but water. It has risen in popularity as a new-age weight loss method, though it has been in existence for thousands of years.

Today, even if you don't consume anything for about 8-12 hours, it is considered fasting. Technically, aren't we all already fasting even though we don't even realize it? A majority of us fast from night until morning when we break our fast. This is exactly why our first meal of the day is called breakfast. Other creatures are always fasting when they get sick. Human beings are probably the only life forms who eat while they are sick despite our bodies signaling us to do otherwise. Therefore, fasting is a normal and integral part of our dietary patterns—it isn't something new. Since primitive times and throughout evolution, our bodies are wired for fasting. Contrary to popular perception, fasting isn't unhealthy or risky if done correctly. It has tons of health benefits.

During the period of water fasting, an individual doesn't consume any other food or drinks. The intake is solely restricted to water, which is believed to facilitate weight loss and good health. Studies have also pointed to the fact that although occasional fasting can benefit short-term weight loss goals, other methods may be more effective in the long run. To ensure you obtain optimal results from your water fasting, prepare well and pick a good time for going without food. Select a time when your body doesn't need a lot of energy if you plan to do water fasting.

There has been plenty of buzz surrounding water fasting as a means of quick weight loss and building a healthy body. It has plenty of benefits—there's no denying that. However, there are also risks attached to it, which we will discuss in detail in the subsequent chapters. Water fasting is believed to reduce the risk of chronic diseases and may trigger autophagy, a physiological process that helps the body break down and recycle old and worn-out parts of your body cells. Though traditionally used for religious purposes, today, water fasting is popular as a natural health and wellness ritual with meditation.

Though there haven't been extensive studies and research on water fasting, it may not be suitable for all. Read everything about the risks attached to it and consult an experienced and qualified medical practitioner before opting for water fasting.

Water fasts have been around for several centuries, though they were practiced using different methods for varying durations (generally 5 to 40 days). The popularity of water fasts has also created several spin-offs on the traditional fasting method. Over the past few years, there have been plenty of offshoots of the original fast—where liquids form the basis of meal plans. Several of these fastings have offered positive results with a decrease in blood pressure.

Though on the face of it, water fasting sounds tough, it can be easier than some other fasting types such as juice or broth fasting. The results can also be much more effective—depending on how and when you do it. Although some people consume black coffee and zero-calorie drinks, these don't qualify for a water fasting. Water fasting is nothing but water.

Water fasting is when you cannot consume anything other than water. A majority of water fasts go on for 24 to 72 hours. Anything longer than this requires medical supervision because it can be dangerous. Some of the most common reasons for water fasting are religious or spiritual purposes, weight loss, detox, health benefits, and getting ready for a medical procedure. Research has connected water fasting with startling health benefits, which is why people are attracted to it. Water fasting is known to lower the risk of heart disease, diabetes, and several forms of cancer. It also facilitates autophagy, as discussed earlier, which helps dangerous and high-risk worn-out cells to be replaced by newer and healthier cells.

Water fasting led to the invention of several other popular diets that were different versions of it—think about the lemon detox method. This version of water fasting allows the person to consume a mixture of cayenne pepper, lemon juice, maple syrup, and water frequently during the day for up to a week.

If you consider the historical perspective, almost every religion suggests some form of fasting—and our ancestors were surprisingly aware of its health benefits, though it may not have been scientifically proven by them. Owing to scarcity, war, famine, floods, and other challenging conditions, people have fasted by default throughout history when they didn't have access to food or during long journeys.

Though today, the thought of going without food seems ridiculous to some people, our ancestors would've probably laughed at the idea of consuming 5-6 meals a day. The 5-6 meals a day concept was totally unheard of before modern times. Therefore, fasting patterns and meal plans evolve a period of time according to the circumstances and conditions prevalent in the era. Though fasting seems ridiculous today, it was once a healthy way of life for erstwhile folks. Now, that people are slowly discovering its benefits—it has made a comeback in a big way.

According to studies that'll amaze you, average Americans do not eat 4-6 meals a day. That's a much conservative figure. The real figure is somewhere near 17-18 times per day. Yes, rub your eyes and read that again. It is 17-18 times a day! You don't think that is possible?

Well, each time you put something that has calories in your mouth, you are creating a digestive event. Even a fistful of nuts, a smoothie sip between meals, or coffee at the end of the day is causing the activation of your body's digestive processes. In short, we end up eating more, moving less, getting less natural sunlight, and exposing ourselves to more artificial light.

We know by now that water fasting leads to autophagy within our bodies. It is nothing but a process of self-eating. Primarily, during autophagy, our body recycles old cells to be replaced by newer and healthier cells. A recent research offers a fitting scientific explanation of autophagy. According to it, autophagy plays a housekeeping role in getting rid of the body's collected proteins, while clearing damaged organelles like endoplasmic reticulum, peroxisomes, and mitochondria. It also eliminates intracellular pathogens. Thus, autophagy is seen as a mechanism of survival.

There have also been studies suggesting that fasting can enhance our digestive health, allowing good bacteria to thrive, which results in an overall increase in the body's metabolic rate, weight reduction, and several other cardiometabolic conditions.

Research reveals that water fasting can help you shed weight by around 14 pounds within five fasting days, reduce blood pressure by an average of 20 points within five fasting days and decrease oxidative stress. Oxidative stress can be defined as a condition characterized by too much oxygen that can play havoc with your body's cells. It is a complex condition—the bottom line of which is that it is an indication that the person is completely out of balance at the cellular level. This condition can lead to increased fatigue, muscle, and joint pain, graying of hair, frequent headaches, noise sensitivity, wrinkles, an ineffective immune system, and poor eyesight.

Let us dive deeper into the subject in order to understand how and why water fasting works while also looking at research studies and debunking some common myths. We'll also discuss other fasting forms to help you pick the one that works best for you.

Chapter One: Stages of Water Fasting

Now that we have some understanding of water fasting, let us understand its physiological effects on the body and how it works. Since no food items or liquids are consumed during the period of water fasting, it can be an intense and strenuous process during which our body gradually learns to adapt to zero food intake. The person doesn't consume anything for energy, which means proper preparation and consultation are vital before one begins fasting. There are multiple periods of adaptation during the fasting period. However, keep in mind that the period before and after fasting is the most important.

Phases of Water Fasting

Water fasting can be categorized into various phases, with each phase having distinct physiological reactions in the body. Let us look at how this form of fasting affects the body during each phase to make for a simpler and more detailed understanding.

Fasting Preparation

Preparing thoroughly for a water fast ensures that your body can slip into the rigors of fasting in a seamless and effortless manner. It helps reduce the stress, anxiety, and shock related to fasting. Before you begin your water fast, prepare yourself mentally for the process. View it as a challenge that needs to be successfully accomplished to fulfill your weight loss and health goals.

Begin by cutting back on your caffeine intake, while also getting rid of added sugar and a variety of dietary fats from your diet a week before you begin your water fast. Avoid consuming processed or preserved foods. Instead, opt for healthier choices such as whole grains, raw vegetables, and fruits. This helps to cleanse the body and gets it geared up for the fast. Again, ensure you speak to a medical representative before deciding to do water fasting for more than five days.

Certain medical conditions can get worse after fasting and could lead to serious health hazards. For purposes of safety, I recommend that anyone interested in water fasting, even those not suffering from any known issues, visit a medical practitioner just to be safe. If you have any of the following conditions, avoid water fasting entirely:

- Alcoholism
- Deficiency of enzymes
- Eating disorders such as bulimia or anorexia
- Liver or kidney ailments (especially in the later stages)
- Dysfunctional thyroid
- Advanced stage cancer
- Diabetes or low blood sugar
- Lupus
- Infectious diseases
- Tuberculosis
- AIDS
- Poor blood circulation or vascular disease
- Paralysis
- Heart diseases and ailments such as valve issues, prior heart attacks, and arrhythmias or cardiomyopathy
- Pregnant or lactating mothers

- Alzheimer's disease
- Post-transplant status
- Being on certain prescription medications

The Fasting Period

The initial six hours following your final meal, your body's glucose, fats, and amino acids will be absorbed as the body digests what was last consumed. Over an initial couple of days, the body starts using glycogen or the accumulated glucose reserve for fueling it. The period lasts for about 12 to 24 hours depending on our metabolism and physical activity. While our body utilizes proteins during the initial fasting week, the amount reduces by half towards the end of the second fasting week. If the fast goes on for over two days, you will go from glycogenosis to ketosis. This is the precise stage where one's liver begins converting fatty acids into ketones, which are substances generated by the body by breaking down fats. These ketones are utilized for fueling the body and muscles. The longer your fasting duration, the longer you will be in the ketosis stage.

Fasting Self-Care

When the fasting period is on, you can't consume foods or liquids other than water, which means your basic intake of water should stay at around six to eight glasses per day. During a water fast, you may be required to drink more than your usual water intake to curb hunger. Also, strenuous physical exertion during a fast isn't recommended. Colon cleanses are popular during water fasts since they facilitate elimination of waste from the system, thus encouraging detox. Water fasts are a good time to undertake your detox regime as the body is effortlessly ready to be cleaned and cleared of all accumulated toxins. According to research conducted by the American Cancer Society, there is no scientific evidence that supports the utilization of enemas and other types of colon therapy, including intake of laxatives.

After Fast

By the end of your fast, you can slowly reintroduce intake of foods over time. Ensure that you don't consume solid foods immediately. This can lead to plenty of discomfort and health ramifications. Go slow and spread it out over a period of time. You may feel hungry owing to the lack of intake of solid foods. However, the plan for reintroducing solid foods is pretty similar for both long and short fasts. Eating a lot of food suddenly will send your digestive system into a state of shock. It has been accustomed to consuming only water for a while. Eating a high-fat and high-protein diet after it has just come out above the rest will shock your digestive system.

Start with raw vegetables and fruits. Fresh juices and clear broths can be especially good. Avoid solid foods for a minimum of three days following the fast. Our body's digestive systems undergo a reverse fasting process. We become more dependent on solid food as the main source of energy over stored fat or protein as we break the water fast. By the fourth day, a person can include whole grains, pulses, and legumes that are well-cooked and soft.

Finally, by the fifth and sixth day, one can start consuming regular meals. One of the most important points to remember while breaking your fast is to keep the body effectively hydrated throughout the process by plenty of fluid intake.

What Happens to Our Body When We Fast?

I am constantly asked if fasting is healthy, and about the physiological processes that happen in our body when we fast. The answer to the former question is that fasting can be increasingly healthy depending on your medical status and how you go about the fasting process. This is exactly why it is highly recommended that you see a doctor before you begin fasting.

When you fast, your body doesn't receive its staple source of energy, which is food. Our liver accumulates plenty of sugar in the glycogen form. This is used as a fallback energy reserve when the body doesn't have any food to dip into. A majority of this energy resource is polished off within the initial 24 fasting hours.

Following this, the body goes into a state known as ketosis. During this particular state, the body's fatty acids act as fuel for replenishing its reducing glucose levels. This usually occurs during the second day of your fast and generally ends by the third day. The body converts glycerol that is available in the body's fat reserves into glucose for obtaining energy. However, this still isn't enough to meet the body's energy requirements. Your body obtains the remaining energy by breaking down amino acids within the muscle tissue, which are utilized by the liver to create glucose to fulfill the body's energy requirements.

After this, ketone production suffices for meeting a majority of the body's energy needs, and the body starts conserving large protein reserves. The body is able to preserve these protein reserves for the protection of muscle tissue and to save important organs from deterioration during long periods without food. For fasts that go beyond a week, the body begins to look for non-body protein fuel reserves. These include among other things, non-essential cellular mechanisms such as degenerative tissues, viruses, and anything the body can use as a source of energy in the absence of new food energy.

Benefits of Water Fasting

Fasting has always been an integral part of our culture for several thousand years, though it has caught the attention of researchers fairly recently. Since there are several therapeutic benefits of fasting being studied every day in modern science, it is important to understand how fasting can impact our overall health and well-being. When you understand the benefits of water fasting, you can use it to your advantage for optimizing your weight loss, anti-aging, and other health goals.

Water fasts can facilitate weight loss.

This is one benefit that a majority of potential fast practitioners are interested in. I am forever asked to share tips on fasting for weight loss. While it seems pretty obvious that staying off food and only drinking water may reduce body fat, it works at a much deeper level than that. Water fasting can help your body reach the ketosis state, where it begins to utilize energy from your internal fat reserves in the absence of new incoming energy sources in form of food. Water fasting facilitates the process of reaching ketosis faster. During this the ketosis state, our body has no option but to break down stored fat cell reserves for energy.

It slows the aging process.

This is another benefit everyone is eagerly interested in. There is no natural known natural force of this planet that can reverse the process of aging (though we've got Botox and a host of other man-made components). Ever wondered why some people are able to slow the aging process while others age faster than you can say Botox? One of the most effective ways of slowing the aging process is fasting regularly. Research conducted on animals has suggested that fasting can increase our lifespan by a maximum of 80 percent. In human beings, fasting has been known to decrease oxidative stress and inflammation.

Enhanced cell recycling

Autophagy is a normal and natural process for replenishing and recycling the body's waste or dysfunctional components. Water fasting causes our body to step into an autophagic stage, which helps restore its dull, damaged and unnecessary cells. With restricted calorie intake, the body is compelled to get into a more selective mode when it comes to protecting its cells. This simply means that fasting can push our body's inherent healing mechanisms into action to destroy, replace and recycle damaged tissues. This can lead to a positive effect on many serious ailments and conditions.

There are many stories about people claiming that water fasting has benefited them in fighting debilitating disorders. There is some research to support these claims though more studies are needed to come to any definite conclusion. Research in animals has revealed that alternate-day fasting can lead to a major decrease in the risk of metabolic syndrome and certain types of cancer. Similarly, rodents put on intermittent fasts revealed lower instances of neurological disorders.

Chapter Two: How to Do a Water Fast?

Honestly, if you ask me, there isn't a more grueling type of fast than a water fast. However, you may not find another fast that is of the same caliber as water fasting in terms of cleansing and detoxifying. It is an inexpensive way of losing weight, focusing on your internal spiritual self and helping your body eliminate its unwanted toxins. Though short-term calorie restrictions can be effective in terms of shedding a few pounds and helping you live a healthier life (if performed correctly), it also has a bunch of risks attached to it. Irrespective of your water fasting goal, it should be done in a safe and appropriate manner by first consulting a healthcare professional. You should also be able to determine when to stop and transition smoothly and gradually to solid foods.

Select the Duration of Your Fast

This is one of the most important considerations before you begin fasting. Begin with a water fast that lasts for a day. You don't want to kill yourself by ambitiously taking on a 5 day fast when your body is just getting accustomed to the idea of going without solid food. If you intend to fast for a longer duration, do it only after getting a go-ahead from an experienced medical practitioner. Fasting retreats are becoming quite popular owing to the fact that those fasting are also under the supervision of medical professionals. It has been noted that fasting for short spans periodically is much safer than going on an extended fast for more than 3 days. Go on a water fast for one day per week.

Also, it is important to note that you mustn't fast during a high-stress period. Schedule your water fast for a time when you won't be under a lot of pressure and stress, which means the fasting won't affect your everyday routine. Whenever it is possible, avoid intense physical work during fasting. Plan your fast for a time when you can be well rested both physically and mentally.

Again, keep in mind that water fasting isn't as easy as it appears on paper. It can be a daunting task when performed practically. Prepare yourself mentally for it by speaking to a medical practitioner/counselor and by talking to people who've successfully done it before. When you view it as a challenge or adventure, you are more likely to enjoy the process, while also deriving health benefits from it.

Do not jump into the fast straightaway, as was explained in the previous chapter. It isn't just plain unhealthy, but can also have tons of risks associated with it. Go slow, and take one step at a time if you want to accomplish your weight loss or health goals with water fasting. Begin eliminating foods such as caffeine, sugar, and processed food items from your diet about 2-3 days prior to the fast. Primarily, stick to vegetables and fruits before the fasting begins.

Another important tip is to reduce your meal portions for several weeks leading up to the fast. This helps prepare your body for the upcoming fast and makes the transition smoother. It makes the overall process much smoother both physically and mentally. Think of using intermittent fasting (more on this later) to lead up to your water fast. You can schedule both types of fasts over the course of a month.

Three weeks before you begin your water fast, stop eating breakfast. During the second week, skip both lunch and breakfast. By the third week, you should be skipping your breakfast and lunch, while reducing the dinner portion. During the fourth week, begin your water fast.

Begin Fast

Consume 9-13 glasses of water a day during your fast. In general, women should consume about 2.2 liters of water a day, while men should consume around 3 liters of water per day. Stick to your daily recommended water intake during the fasting period. Pick the purest and cleanest water you can have, or opt for distilled water.

I know a person who completely misunderstood the water fasting process and drank all the water at one time. Avoid doing this. Instead, spread your water intake throughout the day. Set out three to four one-liter jugs daily to make it easier for you to determine how much water you are consuming in a day. Avoid drinking more than the suggested amount of water as it can throw the salts, minerals, and other nutritious elements in your body for a toss and create health issues. You don't want your essential nutrients washed away by drinking larger than recommended amounts of water.

If you experience hunger pangs, work your way through them by drinking one or two glasses of water. Let the pangs subside and rest. The cravings usually pass after a while. You can also shift your attention to other things or undertake pleasant distractions such as reading, listening to music, and meditating.

Some people experience a sense of dizziness during fasting. This is typically the case after 2-3 fasting days. Avoid this by rising slowly and practicing deep breathing exercises before standing. If you start feeling too dizzy, quickly sit or lie down until the feeling passes. Try to place your head between the knees when it gets a bit too much.

Excessive dizziness can cause you to lose consciousness, which means it's time to stop fasting and see your medical practitioner immediately.

Learn to distinguish between regular and alarming side effects. Some common side effects of water fasting include dizziness, slight weakness, a nauseous feeling, a few skipped heartbeats and so on. However, if you lose consciousness or have heavy heart palpitations for over once or twice a day, it may be time to seek professional medical intervention. Again, severe stomach ache, discomfort, headache, or any other painful or discomfort causing symptom should be addressed immediately. Don't wait for things to get worse. Anything alarming deserves immediate medical attention.

Ensure that you are well rested during the fasting period. There will be a major drop in energy and stamina during the fasting phase, which means you shouldn't exert yourself physically or mentally. Keep a balanced and healthy sleep pattern. Fasting is all about being well-rested – physically, mentally, emotionally and spiritually. Nap each time you feel like taking rest. I'd highly recommend reading inspiring and uplifting spiritual material. Avoid pushing or exerting yourself physically. It is normal to feel tired and out-of-flow. Just give yourself time to relax and rejuvenate.

Your energy levels are constantly fluctuating, which means you end up feeling weak, exhausted, and low on energy. Even if you feel like you have all the energy in the world, avoid taking physically straining yourself. Instead, practice meditation and soft restorative yoga. Intense workouts, cardio, and intense physical activities should be a huge no-no. Yoga is a gentler and subtler alternative if you are looking for light exercise or physical activities. It is a calming and soothing way of moving your muscles and doing some light exercises. While some people will be comfortable practicing yogic postures, others may find them more physically demanding. Don't try it if you haven't done it before. Simply stick to some deep breathing and meditation. The idea is to listen to your body and do whatever makes it comfortable.

While practicing water fasting, it is vital to consume clean, top quality, and fresh water. Contamination in your water will only end up being magnified in the absence of food. Stick to distilled or filtered water during the fast. Filtration can be an option if you have an effective filtration mechanism. However, nothing beats distillation, which goes beyond filtration and eliminated all harmful chemicals and elements from the water.

Organizing a fixed schedule is crucial to the success of water fasting. If possible, consider taking a break from work to cleanse your system during the fast. Choose a fixed duration or for the fast. Though three, seven, and 10 day-long fasts are common, there are people who fast for longer periods. I always recommend beginning small. If this is your first attempt at following a water fast, opt for a 24 hour fast. Three-day fasts are also common for beginners. If you are planning to go on a water fast for more than five days or using it as a way for reducing a serious medical condition, opt for a supervised medical fast. Many people prefer going with a supervised fast since it provides them a more controlled environment along with a team of expert professionals to ensure everything goes smoothly. Plus, you have other fast practitioners for guidance and psychological support.

If you don't know which fast will work best for you, a few tests conducted at a certified fasting clinic can help you with the same. Keep a close check on your health during the fast, and make the transition to solid foods effortless. Let us go over some quick points about fasting precautions. Pregnant and lactating women should avoid fasting, since a developing life is too sensitive to be subjected to nutritional restrictions and deficiencies. Similarly, anyone suffering from Type 1 diabetes should pick different variants of a detox diet. Fasting is more effective for people who weigh over 120 lbs. If you are anything under this, plan a shorter fast if you still want to go ahead and fast, especially if you are fasting for the first time.

Breaking Fast

Break your fast gradually with juices such as lemon and orange. Light broths are also good when it comes to breaking fasts. Later, add foods to your diet slowly. Start with tiny portions every couple of hours, and gradually increase the size of your meals. Proceed in a step-by-step manner from foods that can be easily digested to foods that are tough to digest. Depending on the fast length, the process can be extended over a period of a single day or multiple days depending on how comfortable you are.

Here are some foods in the order which you can consume them while breaking your fast – fruit and vegetable juice, green vegetables and raw fruits, yogurt, cooked veggies and veggie broth, cooked grains, dairy and eggs, poultry (as well as meat and fish). Lastly, everything else!

One of the most important things to remember while going on a water fast is that it won't help much if you get back to consuming a high fat and sugar diet immediately after the fast or even later. Always eat a healthy, nutrition-packed and balanced diet. Consume lots of whole grains, veggies, and fruits. Stick to a diet that is low in unhealthy fats and sugar. Exercise for about half an hour a day for four to five days a week. Maintain a healthy lifestyle to boost your overall health and well-being. Remember, the fasting is only a part of your lifestyle. There are other changes you will need to bring about to make the process of water fasting more effective.

Chapter Three: Intermittent Fasting

Intermittent Fasting (IF) is presently one of the most popular health trends in the world. It is known to have several positive effects on the body such as enhanced health, weight loss, and a more simplified lifestyle. There have been countless studies to point out the benefits of intermittent fasting on the human body and mind.

What Exactly Is Intermittent Fasting?

Intermittent fasting is an eating pattern where a person alternates between periods of eating and fasting. Unlike other diet and meal plans, it doesn't specify what you should eat or avoid. Therefore, it isn't really a diet in its strictest sense. It is more an eating pattern than a conventional diet. Though there are several intermittent methods, some of the most common are daily 16-hour fasts or 24-hour fasts twice a week.

Ancient food gathers and hunters didn't have the convenience of supermarkets and refrigerators. Food wasn't even available throughout the year. At times, they couldn't find anything to eat and went without food for days. The result: through evolution the human body got accustomed to going without food for long durations. I'd go a step further and say fasting is more normal and natural than eating. Fasting is what the body is meant for. Eating more than 3-4 meals may not be as natural for the human body as fasting because our bodies are essentially wired to go without food for longer periods of time. In addition to this, people also fasted for religious purposes. Many religions such as Judaism, Buddhism, Hinduism, and Islam practice going without food for the purpose of cleaning the body and accomplishing other spiritual/religious objectives.

What Are the Different Intermittent Fasting Methods?

Like we discussed above, there are multiple ways to practice intermittent fasting, which involves splitting the 24-hour days of the week into periods of eating and fasting. Different people pick different methods based on what is most convenient or suitable for them. During these fasting periods, you either eat little or nothing.

Here are some of the most popular intermittent fasting methods:

The 16/8 method – The 16/8 intermittent fasting method (also referred to Leangains protocol) comprises skipping breakfast and limiting your daily eating duration to 8 hours. For instance, you may eat from 2 p.m. to 10 p.m. and fast for the remaining 16 hours.

The 5:2 diet – Using this method of intermittent fasting, you focus on consuming merely 500-600 calories on a couple of non-consecutive days within a week. You can ingest regular meals during the remaining 5 days. Reducing calories can be good for weight loss as long as you don't load up on calories during the normal eating periods.

The 5:2 diet is a much sought-after diet plan because it consists of eating for 5 days in a week and limiting calories during a remaining couple of days. The method is also referred to as the Fast Diet and was popularized by doctor-author Michael Mosley. To make the process even more efficient, fasting should be done on nonconsecutive days.

The eat-stop-eat method - This is another popular intermittent fasting method that comprises a 24-hour fasting period once or twice per week. You fast during a 24-hour period. For example, when you eat dinner on Saturday, you don't consume any food until dinner time Sunday, over a 24-hour period. The plan can also be implemented from breakfast or lunch one day until breakfast and lunch respectively until the following day. It doesn't matter whether you begin with lunch, breakfast or dinner as long as you fast over a 24-hour period. Unsweetened coffee, water, and other non-caloric drinks can be consumed during the fast. However, solid food isn't allowed. If you are practicing the eat-stop-eat intermittent fasting plan for the purpose of weight loss, it is important that you eat correctly during your eating window. Consume a healthy, nutritious and balanced meal without starving during your eating window. The only hitch with the eat-stop-eat method is that it can be tough to fast over a 24-hour period, especially if you are not used to fasting.

However, the trick is to get slowly and steadily. Begin with a 13-16 hour fast and then gradually increase the fasting hours until your body gets accustomed to it. When you begin the 24-hour fast, you may feel fine initially but get ravenous towards the end of the fast; this is normal. Fasting like this requires a lot of self-discipline and control. Don't obsess about the timings or be rigid though. If you feel like eating an hour earlier, go ahead and eat. Ensure that you start with something light like a juice or broth and then go back to regular meals.

The warrior diet – The name of this diet evokes an image of a knight on his way to help you combat excess body fat or ill health! The warrior diet was made popular by fitness guru Ori Hofmekler. It involves consuming tiny amounts of raw veggies and fruits during daytime and later eating one large meal for dinner. In short, you limit yourself throughout the day and feast during dinner with a 3-4 hour eating phase. The warrior diet is probably the only intermittent fasting type that focuses on making food choices that are pretty much like the paleo diet comprising unprocessed, whole items that are closest to their natural form.

Spontaneous meal skipping - One doesn't really have to follow a specific intermittent fasting type to enjoy the benefits of the practice. One option is to skip meals and eat whenever convenient. Some people skip meals periodically whenever it is feasible for them. You may want to skip meals when you aren't hungry or too caught up to cook. We'll discuss it in another chapter on fasting myths, but the notion that you have to eat frequent meals or you'll end up starving is a huge myth. Our body is capable of dealing with abstinence from food for extended periods even though we believe fasting is unnatural. Don't fret about getting into starvation mode or losing muscle unless you suffer from a medical condition that requires you to exercise caution while fasting.

If you aren't particularly hungry someday, give breakfast a miss and instead opt for a nutritious lunch. If you are busy throughout the day, leave home after a healthy breakfast and skip lunch to grab a light, well-balanced dinner. I know some people who resort to skipping meals when they can't find anything to eat while traveling. This is probably the best time to go on a mini fast. Skipping a couple of meals whenever you feel like is nothing but a more spontaneous form of intermittent fasting. Ensure that you consume healthy meals at other times though. Also, avoid compensating for calories by overeating during your eating phases.

Beginners find the 16/8 method to be the most sustainable diet plan owing to ease of use and feasibility.

Difference Between Intermittent Fasting and Starvation

I get asked the following question frequently. Isn't intermittent fasting dangerous since it involves starvation?

My answer: no! Intermittent fasting is different from starvation in one important way. The one word for this difference is control. Starvation is involuntary or forced absence from food. It is neither purposeful nor controlled. On the other hand, fasting is the voluntary withholding of meals for spiritual, religious, or health reasons. Food is available but you deliberately choose not to consume it for the stipulated period. It can go on anywhere from a few hours to days to weeks.

Fasting, even if it isn't deliberate, is any period when you abstain from eating. For instance, we all fast by default from dinner until breakfast the next day (unless you are a midnight refrigerator scavenger like one of my friends) for 12-13 hours. Therefore, fasting isn't something new to us. It has always been an integral part of our lives.

How Does Intermittent Fasting Work at a Physiological Level?

So, after all the discussion about what defines intermittent fasting and of the different methods of accomplishing it, let us dive straight into how it works. On a primary level fasting helps your body burn the excess stored fat. Contrary to what many people believe, fasting, when it is done correctly, isn't unnatural or risky unless you suffer from specific medical conditions and have been advised to take caution. The problem is most people are not equipped with the knowledge to fast right.

Let's look at how fasting can be beneficial for the body. Fat is the human body's mechanism of storing energy. When you go without food for extended periods, the body doesn't have any option but to dip into its already accumulated energy reserves stored in the form of fat to meet its energy needs. Think of it like this; what happens when your source of income suddenly comes to a stop? You obviously dip into your savings to meet your daily needs when a consistent income flow stops. Balancing between fasting and eating allows your body to utilize the accumulated fat while maintaining a healthy balance.

When we eat something, the energy that is consumed is not used instantly. A sizeable portion from it is kept in reserve for later use. Insulin, the hormone which is responsible for the body's food storage process, facilitates the process of storing food eaten by us in a couple of ways. Sugar forms a long chain through the glycogen process and is collected in the liver, though it has a limited storage capacity. It can also be transported to deposits elsewhere in the body where there is unlimited storage. The restricted fat storage in the liver is simpler to access than the stored fat in several body parts.

The process then moves into reverse mode while fasting. Insulin levels dip down, and the human body begins to burn accumulated energy because there is no inflow of fresh incoming energy in the body. Glucose levels fall down so the sole way for our body is to burn glucose for meeting its energy needs. Glycogen is the easiest available source of energy, where glucose molecules provide energy to other cells of the body. This process is enough to meet the body's energy supply for 24-36 hours. After that, our body begins to transform stored fat into usable energy.

This means during intermittent fasting, our body exists in dual states, i.e. the feeding and fasting state. In the feeding state, our insulin levels soar, while in the fasting state, they plunge. The human body is forever either storing or burning energy for meeting its energy needs. If the fasting duration is balanced with eating, the body's net weight doesn't increase.

If you are consuming meals from morning to night, we are forever in the eating stage. This means you prevent your body from burning stored fat for meeting its energy requirements. The fat keeps accumulating, without the body using stored reserves (as new sources of energy are available to it). This invariably leads to weight gain since we don't allow our body to get rid of any fat by converting it into energy. To lose weight or maintain body balance, our body needs to burn stored energy, which can happen only by restricting the consumption of food for a specified duration.

One of the most important things to remember about intermittent fasting is that it isn't really harmful. It is about maintaining body function cycles. Like a majority of people, if you are constantly involved in the process of eating, you will continue utilizing the newly incoming food energy without trying to burn what has already been accumulated.

Your body rarely goes into a fasting stage normally. Do you, in general, go on a fast for more than 12 hours between two meals? No, right? This robs your body of the chance to get into the energy-burning process. This is one of the main reasons why folks who practice intermittent fasting release their body fat without making any changes to how much and what they eat, or to their activities. While it is almost impossible to get your body into a fasting state within the standard fasting schedule, intermittent fasting can help fulfill your weight loss and other health goals.

If you begin eating as soon you get out of bed and don't stop until you sleep, you are spending almost all your time in the eating state. Over a period of time, you will keep accumulating the fat energy reserves without offering your body the chance to burn it. When you fast, the body gets enough chances to dip into the stored energy reserves to fulfill its requirements, thus burning accumulated fat and converting it into usable energy for helping you go through your daily activities.

Sudden food withdrawal isn't the best way to get going with intermittent fasting. Researchers and nutrition/diet experts suggest beginning with shorter fasting spans, and progressively increasing them based on your comfort level. You can begin with a 4-8-hour period, and work your way to reaching 12 to 24 hours.

Starting with longer fasting durations can send your non-fast accustomed body into a state of shock, which is not healthy. Give your body the time to get used to going without food by starting with shorter fasting spans. When you feel comfortable fasting for a certain number of hours, slowly increase the number.

However, ensure that you do not go beyond the permissible duration and maintain a healthy balance between fasting and feasting. Give your body time to get accustomed to going without sugar over a period of time. Once it gets into the groove of surviving without sugar for extended periods, increase the fasting duration. This will make it easier for you to fulfill your weight loss and other health goals.

Not everyone's body is the same. If you experience a feeling of tiredness, exhaustion or low energy, switch to a different fasting method. While some people find it challenging to fast on work days but can accomplish their fasting goals during weekends, others find the 16-hour fasting easier. It all depends on your health, fasting objectives, and lifestyle. Which is the most comfortable and convenient intermittent fasting method? No method is perfect. You have to pick the best and make it work to your benefit. Once you practice different methods and gauge their consequences on your body and mind, you are able to make more informed decisions.

Intermittent fasting can be one of the simplest weight loss techniques. It doesn't need much change in your dietary plans and offers great results. This type of fasting is simple to implement and capable of making a huge difference to your weight. Diets may sound easy on the face of it but are often tough to implement. Intermittent fasting is just the opposite. It may seem tough but when you get to it, it isn't really hard to implement.

At its base, fasting lets the body burn excess fat. It is vital to realize that it is normal for humans to fast, and we have fasted over a period of several thousand years without any detrimental effects.

Intermittent Fasting – Points to Keep in Mind Before Fasting

Hunger will be the most common and obvious side effect of any form of fasting. This craving and hunger will come with its fair share of weakness along with the notion that our brain isn't functioning to its optimal capacity.

If you are generally healthy and have a well-nourished body, there may not be any potential risks in going without food for a while. If anything, intermittent fasting regulates, balances, and disciplines your food consumption patterns. However, if you suffer from specific medical conditions that require additional care or are unsure about your body's ability to fast, always speak to a medical practitioner before going on a fast.

People with diabetes, problems regulating blood sugar, eating disorders, fertility problems, low blood pressure, and so on should avoid all forms of intermittent fasting, or fast only after speaking to their doctor. Similarly, pregnant women and lactating mothers should avoid intermittent fasting. People who have a history of anorexia or eating disorders should also stay away from intermittent fasting as it can trigger a resurgence of these conditions.

Also, fasting on specific days shouldn't make you think you can attack high-calorie foods like sweets, junk food, and deep-fried items on eating days. Of course, there will be some reward days (I don't like to call them "cheat days" for some reason; reward days has a more positive ring to it, doesn't it?). However, making every eating period a feast defeats the purpose of intermittent fasting. Keep a close watch on your calorie consumption if you want to lose weight.

Women shouldn't opt for consuming under 500 calories a day, or go without food for a 24-hour period. It can increase stress, and lead to hormonal imbalance. When there is increased calorie restriction, it can play havoc with the menstrual cycle. This is exactly why the 16-8 type of intermittent fasting is believed to the best for women who want to implement it for weight loss or other goals. It is a more feasible and practical plan for women, and one which they can commit to in the long run.

An average intermittent fasting window goes on from 13-17 hours. For people who are just beginning with it, start with giving your breakfast a miss. Then, opt for two meals daily, while maintaining a

7-8 hour eating span. Keep a window of 3-4 hours at least between your dinner and sleep time.

Avoid intermittent fasting if your daily diet consists of processed, artificially sweetened, and tinned food items. The nutritive value of what you eat is integral to the success of your intermittent fasting. Stay away from loading up on unhealthy calories by consuming sugar, refined carbohydrates, and bad fats. Avoid eating junk food and high-carb meals during your eating window. Instead, include more nutritious, protein-packed meals in your diet.

For people who follow a more rigorous and demanding fitness routine, consuming recovery meals is important. Have whey protein around half an hour after your workout. You can try other schedules and meal plans to gauge what suits your fitness regime and objectives the best. Exercise caution while practicing intermittent fasting. Understand your body's requirements and your goals for fasting before going on a fast. Any form of calories restrictions or limitations isn't good for people with diabetes, blood sugar problems, and insulin level issues. Hypoglycemic people should also avoid calorie restrictions.

Intermittent fasting is not an extreme calorie restriction diet, and hence shouldn't be implemented as one. The primary objective of intermittent fasting is to keep a healthy balance between consuming and staying away from calories to keep your body healthy.

The most important thing that several people ignore is that you must feel good about fasting. Yes, this is the single most important factor for success. Other than all the health restrictions, if you do not feel good about fasting, you may want to rework your diet or meal plan. Intermittent fasting should make you feel light, healthy, and positive. If you are forever experiencing feelings of weakness, exhaustion, and crankiness, it may be time to get your act together.

Hunger pangs are normal. A lot of people I know are alarmed by their hunger pangs, which I find slightly amusing. Keep in mind that your body isn't accustomed to going without food for extended durations. There are bound to be some withdrawal symptoms. Stick to a regular fasting schedule once your body identifies the type of fasting that works for it. Avoid changing meal types and fasting types erratically once you are set with a specific fasting routine.

My favorite intermittent fasting survival tip is to manage hunger pangs by consuming black tea or coffee. Minor hunger pangs are natural, and intermittent fasting isn't the same as starving.

As a responsible and well-informed intermittent fasting practitioner, you should understand that there is no magic weapon or secret pill that will help you lose weight overnight. Fat shedding and developing muscle mass happen over a period of time when a healthy diet plan is combined with a healthy lifestyle. Stick to a diet consisting of whole foods and raw vegetables/fruits. Your weight loss toolbox isn't complete without some form of physical activity, workout, or exercise.

Intermittent fasting requires stress reduction mechanisms since you'll tend to feel stressed and low on energy periodically. Practice yoga and/or meditation to eliminate stress and feel more positive throughout the day. Grab sleep for a minimum of 8 hours a day. I know people who lead absolutely unhealthy lifestyles and expect intermittent fasting to be the one pill cure for all their ailments. All your health and nutritional requirements can be met by cutting down on your meals unless otherwise specified according to your medical history. In such a scenario, why complicate things by eating much more than you should?

Benefits of Intermittent Fasting

Here are some benefits or advantages of intermittent fasting:

1. Intermittent fasting alters the function of our cells and hormones.

When you stop eating for a while, there are many changes that happen within your body. For instance, it launches a vital cellular replenishment process and brings about alterations at the hormonal level. This makes accumulated body fat far more accessible. Here are certain changes that happen in our body while we are fasting.

Our blood level insulin drops considerably, which activates the body's fat burning process. In addition to this, our growth hormones' blood levels are significantly boosted (as much as five times the regular levels). Increased level of this hormone expedites the fat burning and muscle gain process, while also having innumerable other benefits. Our body stimulates a vital cellular repair process such as removing scrap material within the cells. Intermittent fasting is also believed to change our genes and molecular make-up to increase our lifespan and offering protection against life-threatening ailments and diseases. Several benefits of intermittent fasting are closely related to transformations in our hormones, genetic expression, and cell functions.

2. It facilitates weight loss and reduction of belly fat.

Many people who practice intermittent fasting do it with the objective of losing weight or blocking off a few extra pounds. It has become a much sought-after weight loss meal plan.

By practicing intermittent fasting, you will eat fewer meals. Unless you compensate by consuming more calories during your eating period, your calorie intake reduces.

Other than this, intermittent fasting boosts the body's hormonal functions to help weight loss. Reduced insulin levels, increased growth hormone levels and a higher amount of non-adrenaline cumulatively facilitate the breakdown of your body's fat reserves and use it for energy to fuel body functions. This is exactly why short-term fasting can boost your body's metabolic rate by 3.6 to 14 percent. Therefore, intermittent fasting is effective on both the sides of this equation. It increases the body's metabolic rate and decreases your food intake. As per a 2014 scientific literature review, intermittent fasting can lead to a weight loss of around 3 to 8 percent over a duration of 3-24 weeks.

3. Intermittent fasting can lower insulin resistance thus reducing the propensity of Type 2 diabetes.

Type 2 diabetes has gained widespread attention in recent years. The most notable feature of Type 2 diabetes is high blood sugar where insulin resistance is concerned. Anything that lowers insulin resistance will reduce blood sugar levels and fight Type 2 diabetes. Intermittent fasting is known to have plenty of significant benefits on the body's insulin resistance and leads to a significant reduction in our blood sugar. In research conducted on humans (thank goodness someone realized our bodies are different from mice) intermittent fasting is known to reduce blood sugar levels by 3 to 6 percent, while insulin (fasting) decreases it by 20 to 32 percent.

One other study conducted on rats (once again rodents made a comeback) suggested that intermittent fasting offers protection against damage to the kidneys, one of the toughest complications arising from diabetes. This simply means that intermittent fasting is great for people who are at a high risk of developing Type 2 diabetes.

4. Intermittent fasting may be beneficial for heart health.

Did you know that the world's number one killer is heart disease? Yes, cardiac ailments consume more lives than anything else, which is why it is important to maintain sound heart health. Several health markers or risk factors are closely connected with either a higher or lower risk of heart ailments. Intermittent fasting has been known to improve innumerable risk factors such as blood pressure, cholesterol, inflammatory markets, and our blood sugar levels. Having said that, much of the research related to the impact of intermittent fasting on heart health has been carried out on animals. The impacts on human health require further research in order to establish a conclusive link between intermittent fasting and heart health.

5. Intermittent fasting can lower oxidative stress and the body's inflammation.

Oxidative stress is one of the main causes of aging and a bunch of chronic ailments. It comprises several unstable molecules termed as free radicals, which get together with other vital molecules to react and damage them. There have been countless studies linking intermittent fasting to a high residence to oxidative stress. Some studies have also revealed that intermittent fasting helps combat inflammation, another cause of common ailments and diseases.

6. Intermittent fasting-induced processes that tackle cellular repair.

When our bodies go on a fast, their cells launch a cellular waste elimination process termed as autophagy (more about its benefits later). During autophagy, the body's cells are broken down and used for metabolizing damaged and dysfunctional proteins that accumulate inside cells through a period of time. Excessive autophagy also fights ailments such as Alzheimer's and cancer.

7. It may help prevent cancer.

Cancer is a life-threatening ailment characterized by uncontrollable cell growth. Fasting impacts our metabolism and may lead to a lower risk of cancer. Although studies conducted within this area are largely confined to animals, there has been an encouraging link between fasting and a longer lifespan due to our body's ability to fight life-threatening diseases. There is also some evidence suggesting that intermittent fasting can help mitigate the harsh effects of chemotherapy.

8. Intermittent fasting is great for brain health.

What is good for the body can be great for the mind and soul too. In the case of intermittent fasting, it is known to enhance our brain health through improved metabolic functions. This includes everything from lower oxidative stress to decreases inflammation to lower blood sugar level along with insulin resistance.

Research conducted on rats has revealed that intermittent fasting is known to boost the growth of new neural cells which can result in a positive impact on our brain functions. Intermittent fasting also boosts brain-derived neurotrophic factor (BDNF), a type of brain hormone. The deficiency of this particular hormone is closely linked with mental conditions such as depression. Again, research conducted on animals had proved pointed to the fact that intermittent fasting fights brain damage arising from strokes.

9. Intermittent fasting may help fight Alzheimer's disease.

Alzheimer's disease is the planet's most widespread neurological ailment. There is no cure for it, which means prevention is the only option for tackling it. Research conducted on rats does point to the fact that intermittent fasting delays Alzheimer's or decreases its intensity. Studies conducted on animals also indicate that fasting offers protection against several other neurodegenerative ailments such as Huntington's and Parkinson's disease.

10. Intermittent fasting boosts your lifespan.

Intermittent fasting may help increase your overall lifespan and help you live longer owing to its ability to prevent the onset of several life-threatening ailments and diseases, including cancer. Research conducted on rats has revealed that intermittent fasting extends our lifespan in a similar manner as prolonged calorie restriction. In one particular study, rats that were made to fast every alternate day survived 83 percent longer than rats who were not subjected to fasting.

Though more studies will be needed to prove this conclusively with regard to humans, Intermittent fasting has become increasingly popular with the weight loss and anti-aging brigade. Given its metabolic effects and a variety of health markers, intermittent fasting can help a person live longer.

11. It is a more positive, feel-good method than other diet plans.

Unlike random crash, unhealthy, and fad diets, intermittent fasting rarely makes you feel low on energy, depressed, or moody. You feel good while practicing it because there is no limit to what you can and cannot eat. There are no start and end dates, unlike other weight loss diets. It doesn't have any fixed duration and can be practiced for as long as you like. In fact, some people have made it an integral part of their lifestyle. As long as you are comfortable and medically fit, you can follow intermittent fasting forever for weight loss, maintaining muscle mass, and health purposes. Unlike other starvation-based diets, you look and feel greater after following intermittent fasting.

Generally, people who follow intermittent fasting regularly do not feel drained or tired forever. Our energy levels rise because we are eating in a more purposeful and balanced way. Another aspect where intermittent scores are that instead of approaching eating as just another chore to be fulfilling, you get into the habit of eating in a more mindful and appreciative way. If you combine fasting with increased physical activity or a regular fitness regime, you can witness even more splendid weight loss results, if that's your main goal for fasting.

One of the best parts about intermittent fasting that attracts plenty of people to it, in my opinion, is that it isn't as challenging or demanding as dieting. We've all seen New Year's resolution diets crash during the first week of January owing to low resolve and challenging application. Though fancy weight loss and healthy diets look pretty good in a book filled with facts and pictures, they are tough to implement in the real world, especially for people who lead a busy life. Diet plans can be tough to accommodate in your daily lifestyle. Unless you are a celebrity with 20 assistants running around you and sourcing your food, where on earth will you get some rare type of food that is exactly as per your dietary specifications? Diet plans are not really feasible because you don't have access to certain types of foods wherever you go unless you carry your tiffin around like a school child. Hence, it is not convenient to sustain diet plans in the long run.

On the contrary, intermittent fasting can be easily included into your everyday life. The practitioner doesn't have to stick to specified food groups or kinds of food. You have the convenience, ease, and flexibility to eat anything that is easily available as long as the total number of calories is not alarmingly high. There is greater flexibility about when you want to fast and eat, based on your lifestyle and everyday schedule. Unlike fad diets, intermittent fasting doesn't leave you exhausted, angry, and hungry. There is little stress about what to eat and avoid.

Now I am not suggesting that intermittent fasting is the easiest thing you'll ever follow on the planet. It will obviously take time for your body to adapt to the new eating patterns. A lot of new practitioners do experience "teething pains" when it comes to getting their bodies used to the idea of staying without food for several hours at a stretch. I loved my food, and couldn't imagine the idea going without it for hours at a time. If you'd asked me to follow intermittent fasting in my younger days, I'd have laughed hard. But here I am today – happy, glowing and enjoying the benefits of intermittent fasting. The reason why I am sharing this is to offer you hope that you aren't alone. There will be days when you'll feel like you won't be able to go without food for another second. Develop a coping mechanism for such days. At times, it is alright to break your resolve and eat a couple of hours earlier if you are feeling really weak and hungry. There are no rules set in stone regarding what you can and cannot do. The fast is for your body, and your benefit. If you find that it does more harm to the body rather than helping it, change the way you do things or opt for a different fasting plan. The bottom line is that you should feel wonderful about fasting at the end of the day.

During intermittent fasting, you can continue eating the foods you normally eat provided you don't eat a lot of unhealthy food regularly, and your total number of calories isn't too high.

I want you to do a small 5-10-minute activity that will help you understand the difference between intermittent fasting and other diet plans. Do a quick search on Google to find out the season's latest and most popular diets and weight loss trends. In the majority of cases, you'll come up with a list of diets, each one with its own big list on the type of foods to eat and avoid. Each will most likely have a complicated checklist, a range of cookbooks, and a rigid list of dos and don'ts to follow.

There are no specific recipes or overpriced instructional cookbooks for fasting. You don't have to work with a list of forbidden and permitted foods. Of course, you will have to follow smarter, healthier, and more mindful eating practices such as sugar reduction, avoiding artificially sweetened foods, and packaged meals to experience effective weight loss. There aren't any special types of food items or meal preparation methods involved. If you consume balanced, low calorie, and nutritious meals, while also cutting back on processed and junk food, there isn't an endless list of restrictions. What I enjoy most about intermittent fasting is that you can consume everything in moderation.

Much like other diets and meal plans, intermittent fasting isn't simply related to weight loss. It runs deeper than that. It is about building healthy food consumption patterns, regulating your food habits, building greater muscle mass, and flaunting a more well-built or toned physique. Of course, weight loss objectives are closely linked with intermittent fasting. However, on the whole, it is about accomplishing your weight loss and health goals in a healthy, disciplined, determined and balanced way.

12. Intermittent fasting simplifies your lifestyle.

Irrespective of how proud you are of your cooking and meal planning skills, there's no denying that cooking is a time-consuming, cumbersome, and tedious process. Creating a menu, planning meals, preparing food, packing meals, and cleaning up can be arduous if done every day. Life can get much simpler (and I say this from first-hand experience) when you are dealing with lesser and lighter meals. You can focus on tasks other than planning meals, and picking up ingredients for 3-4 meals a day.

For example, let us assume that you are on the 16-8 intermittent fasting plan. If you skip lunch, all that needs to be done is consuming a healthy breakfast before leaving home or beginning with your daily chores. This can be followed by calorie-free tea or coffee throughout the day and planning a light nutritious dinner. You are removing an entire meal from the day, which means less planning and cooking to simplify your life.

Not just that, amusing as it sounds, you'll also end up saving a lot of money by skipping some meals. Eat fewer meals in quantity, but higher in quality in terms of nutrition and balance. You'll save on plenty of time that would have been spent cooking, grocery shopping, and meal planning: time which can be better utilized by practicing some form of physical fitness to supplement your fast and by leading a more disciplined lifestyle. Further benefits will include your glowing appearance and the loads of compliments you will receive!

13. It establishes a clear eating routine.

Be honest while answering this, how many of us really eat at a fixed time every day? We've all been guilty of being too busy with work and grabbing a sandwich at 3 p.m. or dashing off without eating breakfast or digging into our favorite midnight snack when hunger pangs strike. Truth is, unless we follow a specific eating pattern, we will forever test the limits of our body until it decides to snap and results in a host of health issues. We skip meals to meet deadlines or go without food for hours while preparing for that all-important presentation. We know it isn't healthy for our bodies. However, at some point or another, we've all done damage to our body by not eating at a fixed time each day. Intermittent fasting lets you set fixed meal consumption and fasting hours to streamline the process of sticking to a regular eating schedule. This is also wonderful from the health and weight loss perspective. You can plan your routine and work around when you are likelier to feel hungry or satiated. This can be highly convenient when it comes to scheduling your everyday activities. Once you know you will be fasting during certain times, it is easier to reserve your fasting period for less strenuous activities.

14. Intermittent fasting is highly beneficial for athletes.

Though there are extensive discussions and debate surrounding the benefits and drawbacks of intermittent fasting for sportspersons, it isn't too far-fetched to say that its benefits for regular practitioners are also applicable to athletes or people engaging in intense physical activities or tasks.

Fasting sportspersons can witness several benefits of intermittent fasting like increased growth hormones, reduced inflammation, detox, and low-calorie intake. Day-long fasts are known to be effective when it comes to recovering from aches and minor injuries. For athletes who want to control their weight, regulate their fat levels and maintain muscle mass, fasting can spell good news.

Here are some tips to help sportspersons maximize the benefits of intermittent fasting for boosting their performance on the field:

1. Opt for longer feeding phases than regular practitioners because you may require higher calorie intake for recovering from the strain, physical training, and injury. Reduce fasting windows to around 4-8 hours.

2. Avoid cutting back on calories. Yes, intermittent fasting for weight loss involves going easy on calories. However, when you are eating fewer meals, it is vital for the body to keep a healthy calorie count to meet your strength training, recovery and intense physical activity goals.

3. Intake more proteins as will help control your food cravings during the fasting window. Your cravings reduce, and you'll notice a greater sense of fullness of satiation. How does this happen? Amino acids in proteins help you stay positive, alert and focused while keeping on track (literally and figuratively).

4. Eat at the same time each day. Avoid following spontaneous or erratic intermittent fasting by eating and skipping meals whenever you feel like. It may work for some people but isn't suitable for athletes or people who are engaged in high-intensity physical activities. Establish a regular eating schedule for all days to balance cortisol levels and optimize maximizing rhythms for improving on-field performance.

5. Avoid fasting during high-intensity competitions and training. Fasting for athletes isn't recommended when they are undertaking high-intensity training, participating in high-pressure competitions, or undergoing volume training. Depriving your body of calories needed to fulfill its nutritional and replenishment requirements during a performance isn't a good idea.

6. Restrict consumption of caffeine – Though it is fine to start your day with some coffee for surviving food cravings until lunchtime, it is a good idea to keep sipping on it each time you experience hunger pangs. Excessive coffee consumption can lead to an imbalance in your brain's cortisol levels, thus making you feel more stressed and mentally exhausted.

7. Fasting experts and researchers recommend that athletes should stick to low-intensity workouts such as cardio while in their fasting window. On the other hand, high-intensity workouts or endurance training should be reserved for eating phases or days.

8. Bear in mind that fasting makes the process of building muscles by endurance training and the resulting weight loss tougher in the long run. This is due to the fact that burning protein has a direct effect on your muscular strength and slows down your metabolism over a period of time. However you practice intermittent fasting, it

isn't going to make dramatic changes to your eating pattern, especially if your body is not accustomed to fasting. Follow any intermittent fasting plan only after doing proper research (according to your body's needs and your fasting goals), sticking to a well-planned, nutrition rich and balanced diet, and consulting a doctor. Take into account your physiological and psychological needs before picking a fasting plan.

Disadvantages of Intermittent Fasting

While intermittent fasting has several benefits, much like any other eating or diet plan, it also comes with its share of shortcomings. On the whole there may be more advantages than disadvantages, but it is still important to run through the negative points to make more informed choices. Here's a quick look at some of the disadvantages of intermittent fasting.

Intermittent fasting may cause lead to eating disorders.

This can happen only when it is practiced without moderation in unhealthily extreme forms. Intermittent fasting can cause eating disorders like binge eating and purging. Likewise, it can lead to overeating or anorexia, which turn can cause a bunch of other psychological issues such as feelings of guilt or shame over time. Don't fast for unhealthy reasons or take it to extreme levels. Ensure you are eating well-balanced and nutritious meals during your eating phase. Avoid obsessing over calorie intake and instead focus on making smarter food choices.

All types of fasting, intermittent or otherwise, are best avoided by people with a history of eating disorders or emotion-driven eating patterns. It can trigger the condition again and increase already existing psychological issues. If you are presently in a more negative frame of mind or psychologically stressed/disturbed, it may not be the best time to fast. Wait until you are in a more positive frame of mind to start with your intermittent fasting plan. Fasting during a psychologically stressed period can lead to greater hormonal imbalances, and end up worsening your condition.

Unhealthy obsession with food

Let us assume you've been fasting for 10 hours now throughout the day, and a friend just opens a box of delicious takeaway. What is your reaction? Fasting can increase your obsession with the idea of eating your next meal and food. The focus often shifts from all other pursuits onto when your fasting hours will be over. The tendency to watch the clock and wait for the next meal can interfere with your day to day activities if you make it an unhealthy obsession. If fasting governs all your other activities and lowers your productivity, it may not be so beneficial after all. Don't let eating occupy center stage while all other activities are placed on the backburner. Make smart food choices, follow the survival tips mentioned in this book, and most importantly – don't starve yourself. All this can create an unhealthy obsession with fasting.

Excessive dependence on caffeine

If you are going to function without food for 15-16 hours per day, you will need tea or coffee to keep hunger pangs and food cravings in check. This will lead to an increase in caffeine consumption over a period of time, especially during the fasting window. Several practitioners have a tendency to use coffee or tea as a quick fix for keeping themselves charged throughout the fasting phase. It may be the only way for some individuals to survive without eating for extended periods. However, this increase in caffeine consumption can have several repercussions, the most notable being disturbed sleep patterns, anxiety, stress, mood swings, and depression.

Caffeine is known to boost the body's cortisol levels (our body's stress causing hormones). Even a small increase in our cortisol levels can cause our blood sugar level to shoot up and increase insulin resistance. Thus, getting addicted to caffeine as a side effect of your intermittent fast plan is not a good idea.

Fasting can cause food intolerance.

Fasting can leave a person physically and mentally drained. This can trigger eating binges during your eating phase. Once you load up on calories after a long gap, your calories as well as sugar increases and crashes, thus creating even more prominent hunger pangs and food cravings. If your first post-fast meal consists of more reactive food items in greater quantities, it can cause massive food intolerance with conditions such as inflammation. This, in turn, can increase the risk of Type 1 diabetes. Inflammation is also known to be one of the most common causes of weight gain in the United States of America.

Malnutrition

Any type of fast comes with the dangers of malnutrition. There may be a good chance that you are not fulfilling your body's nutritional requirement by not consuming the right type of food. Intermittent fasting comprises reducing calorie consumption and consuming meals, which means if you don't make smart eating choices you could end up eating meals that are low in nutrition. This can lead to low blood pressure, nausea, and mouth dryness. Since our body's calorie consumption has been reduced, it automatically plunges into survival mode, thus reducing our body's overall metabolism, lowering energy levels and general stamina for performing physical activities. It can lead to a perpetual feeling of being exhausted and stressed, which in turn can impact your personal and professional life.

Fasting may increase stress.

Fasting keeps our body's cortisol stress hormones in control, focusing on existing active adrenals. Research has suggested that fasting for 48 straight hours boosts our cortisol levels, thus leading to the idea that intermittent fasting (especially over an extended period) can lead to increased stress and a general feeling of mental tiredness. Even if you don't undergo fasting for long but have a history of fatigue or stress-related conditions such as depression or anxiety, fasting may end up worsening it.

Frequently Asked Questions About Intermittent Fasting

Q. Is intermittent fasting suitable for women?

I've been frequently asked if intermittent fasting is indeed suitable for women. There is evidence pointing to the idea that it may not be as advantageous for women as it is for men.

For instance, one study indicated that intermittent fasting enhanced brain insulin sensitivity in men, though it reduced blood sugar regulation in women. Though there is no access to human studies regarding this, research of female rats has revealed that fasting makes them more infertile and leads to missed menstrual cycles. There are several unconfirmed reports suggesting that intermittent fasting interferes with a woman's menstrual cycle, and that normal cycles will resume only when the fasting stops.

For precisely these reasons, women must exercise some caution while going on an intermittent fast. This isn't to say that they shouldn't fast or that intermittent fasting is absolutely unhealthy for women. It only suggests that they should be more careful, read up about the effects of fasting, and consult a medical practitioner to make more informed choices. Follow some guidelines such as stopping intermittent fasting immediately in the event of issues such as amenorrhea or missed menstruation. For women who are grappling with fertility issues, it is best to avoid intermittent fasting for the time being. Intermittent fasting is also a bad idea for pregnant and lactating women. Again, women with a history of eating disorders, depression, emotional issues, and psychological ailments should stay away from fasting. Additionally, intermittent fasting may be bad news for underweight women.

There is plenty of discussion about the consequences of intermittent fasting on the female body. While some experts are of the view that fasting has a direct impact on a woman's fertility, there isn't really concrete evidence to support this. More research on humans is required to shed light on the topic. Keep in mind that anything done in extremes is not good for your health, which also holds true for intermittent fasting. Fasting for over 24 hours is not recommended as it can cause detrimental side effects. Intermittent fasting may also lead to hormonal imbalances while impacting your body's ability to conceive.

Ideally, women shouldn't go on prolonged. Try to practice intermittent fasting for shorter durations to avoid playing havoc with your hormones. Some amount of metabolic change shouldn't set off your alarm bells. It may not affect your menstrual cycle in the long run. An average healthy woman may not really experience any visible side effects where menstruation is concerned unless you are doing it in excess or fasting beyond regularly feasible limits. Avoid starving yourself for extended periods or consuming unhealthy meals during your eating window and you should be fine.

Intermittent fasting experts do not suggest fasting when you are stressed or in an emotionally imbalanced state as it can cause further trouble or aggravate the psychological condition, which can further hormonal imbalances. It may be an instance of fasting under not so favorable circumstances, leading to several side effects which may not occur in normal circumstance. There is no clear evidence to directly link intermittent fasting with fertility and menstrual issues. Ensure that you don't do fasting for more than 24 hours.

If you are fasting for more than 24 hours, avoid doing it for over twice a week. Similarly, you can also begin by practicing the much easier and feasible 16-8 intermittent fasting plan. According to some studies, women witness better results by fasting for shorter durations than men.

However, looking at the bigger picture, intermittent fasting is known to be more beneficial for men—though women can follow it by sticking to health and safety guidelines.

Q. Does intermittent fasting lead to a state of starvation?

We've all visited fancy department stores that sell among a range of other items, things such as apparel, footwear, and accessories. Let us examine the concept of intermittent fasting and what it does to the body based on this widely understood analogy. When you visit a department store, there is a range of products on display on a rack for buyers to purchase.

However, there is also another inventory somewhere in the warehouse or storeroom that is in line to go on racks once the items on the racks are sold off. There are a limited number of products that can be displayed on the racks or shelves. The additional merchandise, therefore, has to be stocked elsewhere in a warehouse. There is always new stuff being added to the product inventory, thus filling the warehouse. Brand new seasonal collections are forever making their way into the warehouse. Now, the stuff on shelves is also being sold rapidly. All of a sudden, the store decides not to include any new inventory owing to business decisions. Do you think you'll walk into the store to find empty shelves and racks? No way! There will be tons of merchandise still waiting to be picked up. There is a lot of stuff still waiting to be sold in the warehouse, isn't there? Even when the store has decided to halt its process of sourcing new products or adding to the product inventory, there are tons of products stocked in the warehouse, waiting to be sold. Instead of keeping the racks and shelves empty, the products in the warehouse will be quickly put on shelves.

Now use the exact logic when it comes to the body. Glucose is your body's staple short-term energy provider (think products on the shelves or rack), while fat is the long-term energy provider (think inventory stocked in the warehouse). Fat won't be utilized or burned when the body has glucose to fuel its energy, just like the stocked warehouse inventory will not be put on racks until the inventory on the racks remains unsold.

When glucose resources are immediately available to the body, it will utilize it and not touch the fat. What happens when the body doesn't have any glucose left for further use? It doesn't starve much like the store's racks and shelves aren't left empty. There is still a steady supply of fat waiting to be burnt for meeting the body's energy requirements. The body goes around accumulating stored fat, which will be used in for energy when glucose is unavailable to the body. This means that the body rarely starves unless you fast for a really long time. Our body is wired for intuitively identifying and adapting to diverse energy resources in the absence of glucose. Fat energy or items stored in the warehouse are released when the glucose quota completely depletes.

Q. Is consuming beverages and/or juices allowed during intermittent fasting?

This is another question that is raised frequently by people wanting to try intermittent fasting. They worry about how they'll be able to sustain the fasting phase and if they can keep themselves going with juices and beverages.

The answer is, you can consume calorie-free coffee, green tea and water during the fasting phase to control hunger pangs. Sparkling water is another good option for those looking for zero calorie drinks. At times, low-calorie drinks are also fine though you should avoid fancy coffee shop frills such as cream, artificial sweeteners, and chocolate. You will only load up on unnecessary calories. Even when you are going out for social gatherings or partying, it helps to make and carry your own beverages rather than depending on vending machines and cafes. Avoid calorie filled artificial sweeteners and dairy.

Also, juices are not completely calorie-free and are generally not advisable during the fasting phase though they are a good option to break your fast with. It all boils down to your individual goals for fasting. If you are fasting to lose weight, then you may want to zero-calorie drinks only. However, some people also like to consume low-calorie drinks to help them sustain through the fasting period. Whatever rocks your boat as long as you don't overdo it and stick to the general intermittent fasting framework!

If you go on a 24-hour fast, there may be some sweet cravings especially if you just can't do with your desserts. You do not just need nutrition but also a determination to tide through this phase. In such a scenario, opt for fresh homemade veggie and fruit juices. They should ideally be free from artificial sweeteners as well as added preservatives. Have them without sugar to allow the body some nourishment, sustenance and a sense of fulfillment for sweet cravings.

Also, keep drinking water in unlimited amounts throughout the fasting phase to keep your body sufficiently hydrated during the fasting phase. Going without water for long can be even more harmful when you are fasting because your body doesn't intake water from any other food substances. It will help in preventing conditions such as brain swelling, sunstroke, and kidney malfunctioning.

I also recommend infused water during the fasting phase. Just keep water in a tumbler and add a dash of lime to it. It'll pack more punch in your drink and also help cleanse or detox your body. Lemon water is refreshing, especially if you are feeling dehydrated or low on energy. You can also drink vegetable stock after you finish boiling your veggies in it. Just add some salt and pepper, and you're good to go. It is delicious, wholesome and easy to digest. These are creative ways to intake water when it gets too boring. These light, easy and refreshing drinks can help keep hunger at bay during your fasting phase. Add natural flavors and elements to make your liquids more interesting.

Q. On an average, how many calories should a person consume while following the intermittent fasting plan?

The answer is, it depends on your unique and individual objectives for fasting. What are your fasting goals? If weight loss is the fundamental goal, how many pounds do you want to knock off? How is your body's metabolism? There is no prescribed calorie intake recommended in intermittent fasting unless you are specifically opting for a calorie-based variant of intermittent fasting, where you are expected to limit your meals to a stimulated number of calories. Other than that, if you are opting for a regular intermittent fasting plan such as the 16-8 type, there are no calorie intake specifications. As a rule of the thumb though, keep your calorie intake within 1000-2000 calories/per day, more so if you are fasting with the objective of losing weight.

Rather than obsessing about your calorie intake, I would suggest focusing on eating balanced, wholesome and nutritious meals. Consume everything in moderation to maintain an active and healthy lifestyle. Regulate your meal eating patterns to fulfill weight loss goals through intermittent fasting. Reducing your calorie intake is just one component of the plan. There are several other things like exercising or leading a more physically active lifestyle. Don't turn into a bundle of calorie counting nerves before every meal. Instead, concentrate on lowering your intake of sugar and processed food. Make healthier food choices by opting for fresh, whole and high fiber foods.

Bid adieu to artificially sweetened, processed, and canned food products. Again, on the whole, avoid consuming aerated drinks. I know people who go on erratic, knee-jerk diet plans and completely deprive their bodies of calories, which is not the best way to do it. Sudden deprivation of calories may not be healthy for the body. It will only increase your food cravings and lead to unhealthy physiological effects in the long run. Instead of obsessing over curbing calorie intake, focus on consuming protein-rich and fibrous meals. Stay away from harmful carbs and bad fats to meet your weight loss and other intermittent fasting objectives.

Q. Does intermittent fasting lower the body's metabolism rate?

This is not true and originates from the viewpoint that eating directly affects our metabolism. Eating doesn't directly affect our body's metabolic rate. It influences it through a process known as thermal feeding. The human body is perpetually spending energy for the purpose of performing several functions such as digestion and food absorption. This is the only connection used to conclude that by not consuming food, we are affecting or slowing our body's metabolic rate. It is a mistaken notion that eating light meals frequently increases the body's metabolism levels.

Our body's thermal effect is determined by the overall consumption of energy and not our food consumption frequency or intervals of breaking down the body's consumed calories. You can once or twenty-five times a day and still intake the same number of calories based on what you are eating. You can eat a single meal of 1200 calories or break it into six meals of 200 calories. Bottom line – the overall calorie consumption stays the same. The body's overall metabolism remains unaffected if you phase out your eating over a given period instead of consuming all calories at once.

Q. Can I take any supplements to simplify the process of fasting?

Similar to other weight loss and diet plans, you can take nutritional supplements while following the intermittent fasting plan. However, ensure you consult a medical practitioner, certified nutritionist or dietician before you opt for nutritional supplements to complement your intermittent fasting plan. Irrespective of your goal, you have to ascertain that your body's nutritional needs are fulfilled in a balanced and healthy manner. You may want to consider taking a multivitamin supplement daily. Fish oil supplements are can also be considered. Then there are Amino acids and Vitamin D supplements, which are fairly common with intermittent fasting practitioners.

If you also plan to stick to a fitness regime, amino acids may be a good option. After consulting with a nutritionist or medical practitioner, they can be consumed pre and post your workout to facilitate the body's energy gain and muscle stain reduction process. Folks who suffer from fluctuating moods and other psychological ailments such as depression, bipolar and obsessive-compulsive disorder are also believed to use BCAA supplements for fighting a general feeling of grumpiness, hopelessness, and depression during the fasting period.

Top Mistakes People Make While Practicing Intermittent Fasting

So, you've seen your favorite viral site feature this fasting method which is currently a rage among the Hollywood brigade and shows no sign of dwindling on the popularity meter and decided to jump on the bandwagon to enjoy its weight loss and other health benefits. Well, as I mentioned before, it is beneficial only if you do it right.

There are plenty of people who jump into it without consulting health professionals or knowing what is best for them. Your best bud may have knocked off 20 pounds, and your uncle may have regulated his blood sugar levels through intermittent fasting. However, when you try it yourself, there are zilch results. Here is a compilation of some of the most common and biggest blunders people make when following an intermittent fasting regime.

1. You're going at breakneck speed, buddy.

Hold on and go easy. The most reason for the failure of most diets is that they are considerably far-fetched from our regular eating or food consumption routines. It feels almost impossible to maintain them in the longer run. Throwing yourself into hardcore 24-hour intermittent fasting won't work if you are accustomed to eating tiny meals every couple of hours. Start with a more practical beginner's 12-12 fast, where you are eating for 12 hours and fasting for the remaining 12 hours. This is more practical because it comes closer to what you've already been following until now. It can be more sustainable in the long. When you feel more comfortable, gradually increase the fasting duration.

Our bodies are not accustomed to erratic eating (unless you don't have fixed meal schedules) or going without food for long durations. If you make it do too much too soon, it will give away and snap. You don't want to send your body into a shock as soon as you begin, and then end the fast before you can even say intermittent fasting. That's not how it should work. If you want to sustain with your intermittent fasting plan, in the long run, go slow and steady. Take one step at a time to see how your body reacts to it. Give your body the time to get used to going without meals for longer durations than it is currently accustomed to. Eventually, it will come around and respond favorably to the fasting plan. You will feel much more positive, healthy and energetic when you take gradual steps while following the fast.

2. Not picking a plan that suits your lifestyle

Sue from five blocks away may have lost 15 pounds and looks stunning as hell by following the 8-16 intermittent fasting method. However, this doesn't mean the plan will automatically work for you too. Your lifestyle may be different from that of Sue, which means you have to pick a diet plan that is appropriate for your unique lifestyle.

Take into account your physical activity regime, professional life, household responsibilities and more into consideration before picking a plan that is most suitable for you. Don't opt for a mismatched diet that is a plan from hell. For example, it doesn't make sense to begin fasting at 7 p.m. if you are a night bird. Similarly, gym ninjas should avoid fasting methods that considerably limit their calorie intake if they are following a heavy-duty exercise routine. Weave your diet plan seamlessly into your lifestyle to accomplish best results.

3. Overeating during the eating window

Now, what is the point of consuming double the number of calories during your eating window to compensate for the fasting phases? The trick is not to starve yourself so much that the minute the clock ticks to your eating time; you eat with gusto. If you can't go without food for extended periods, do not pick a highly restrictive regime.

According to studies, restrictive diets often fail because we tend to get physically and emotionally starved, and when we are allowed to eat, we go all out and hog. Maintain a less rigorous diet if you can't sustain increasingly restrictive diets in the long run.

4. Not eating well during the eating phase

Not eating sufficiently is the opposite of the third point. It can also be a factor contributing towards weight gain. Apart from positioning yourself for the rebound as discussed above, not consuming enough food during the eating phase cannibalizes our muscle mass, and causes the body's metabolism rate to reduce. Without muscle mass, you can sabotage your body's ability to store (forget about losing) fat in the future.

The tricky part about intermittent fasting is that you tend to eat according to arbitrary rules instead of listening to your body's natural clues. It is tough to understand your body's real needs. Don't do anything that makes your body feel uncomfortable or unnatural, and always consult a registered dietician to cover your nutrition and safety needs.

5. Trying to do too many things at once

Yes, you think you possess the force and power of all superheroes put together, which makes you under eat, fast and train excessively. If you have spent several days not eating well or avoiding a regular exercise routine, don't attempt to swallow more than you are able to chew- literally right in the beginning. Slip yourself into a fasting regime and training slowly. Avoid beginning training five times a week or fast daily. It'll get too much for you to handle. The result can be adrenal fatigue. While our body is habituated to some form of stress, stretching it to test its limits is a bit too much.

6. Increased obsession with eating windows and fasting-eating timing

You may have landed straight from the military but there's no reason to be obsessed with eating windows and the fasting-eating timing. Align with your body and learn to identify real hunger that strikes every 15-24 hours and not every couple of hours. Allow your body and not the clock to determine when you should be eating. If you are forever looking at the clock, you are doing nothing but counting hours when you can attack food again with gusto. Learn to respond to your body signals instead.

For instance, let's say you are opting for the 2 Meal Day and opt to miss either breakfast or dinner, and plan to extend your overnight fast to around 16 hours. Don't obsess over the time duration. Instead, if you opt to skip breakfast, eat when you feel hungry. Listen to your body and customize/tailor your fast according to your body's unique needs instead of simply going by the clock to the tee.

Listening to your body signals may offer you more effective results over rigidly sticking to eating and fasting windows. As long as you are following the basic framework and principles of the fast, it is alright to tweak it a bit here and there. Remember, you are not making any major changes. Instead, you are responding to your body's needs and aligning your habits with your unique system.

Don't sacrifice what you eat for your obsessive quest with "when." Intermittent fasting as such is a time focused diet. A majority of diets have explicit rules about what you can and cannot consume. However, intermittent fasting doesn't tell you what you can or cannot eat during your eating phases. Don't make that your excuses for feasting on French fries, sinful milkshakes, and double-cheese loaded pizza. Fasting doesn't create miracles. It brings about tiny metabolic changes within the body. However, its fundamental impact on weight loss is considerably based on restricting the number of eating hours to reduce calorie consumption opportunities. You are lowering your hours of eating because you want to decrease the number of calories consumed per day. If you load up on calories during your eating window, the main principle behind fasting is totally defeated.

Don't make intermittent fasting a reason for eating rubbish. It can be a highly effective method for controlling your weight and overall health. However, it doesn't cancel the effect of consuming processed, high-fat and sugar-rich foods. It is even more important to provide proper nutrition to your body when you are fasting. Therefore, stick to whole foods that are high in nutritive value. When our bodies are in the fasting state, it means we are increasingly sensitive to the food we consume. This is wonderful if you are sticking to a nutrition-packed meal. If you are not nourishing your body with rich nutrients, your body will keep craving nourishment, which will invariably lead to frequent hunger pangs (something you don't really want during your fasting phase).

You can immediately the undo the effect of all your hard work in by opting to eat the wrong types of foods. I know some people who operate with the belief that the eating window is their time to treat themselves for having survived without food for long. It doesn't work like this, unfortunately. Instead of viewing your hours for eating and feasting, see it as the time to load up on nutrition rich food. Ensure each meal you consume is packed with high fiber, healthy good fats, and protein. These high nutrition foods will allow you to sustain throughout the fasting window. There's a trick to do it right, and I've shared almost all of them here.

7. Not drinking sufficient water

I know a lot of you don't think this is a big deal. However, when your body is in the fasting state, it begins breaking down damaged and destroyed components and detoxifies our body. It is vital for harmful toxins to be flushed out of our body, which is why drinking a minimum of 4-5 liters of water daily should be a must. One of the best tips for feeling full during the fasting window is to keep sipping on sparkling water. It helps you feel experience a feeling of fullness even on an empty stomach, thus allowing you to sustain the fast over its stipulated period.

Remember, your intermittent fasting regime restricts you from consuming food, not water. You should as much water as you can. This becomes even more important because your body is missing hydration derived from fresh fruits and vegetables. Dehydration can lead to several ailments and discomfort causing conditions such as headaches, hunger pangs, cramps and so on. Ensure you are forever sipping on water during fasts. No excuses.

Chapter Four: Alternate Day and Extended Day Fasting

Alternate-Day Fasting

Alternate-day fasting is nothing but a type of intermittent fasting. With this meal plan, you fast every other day. However, there are no restrictions on what you can consume on non-fasting days. The most widespread version of alternate-day fasting comprises "modified fasting," where you limit your calorie intake to 500 calories/day on fasting days. Alternate fasting is another powerful fasting method known to possess plenty of health benefits such as a lower risk of heart ailments and Type 2 diabetes.

Want to know more about alternate-day fasting? Here's the detailed insider information you are looking for.

As is evident from its name, alternate fasting is about switching between consuming regular meals one day and consuming 25 percent of calories the next day. There are several versions of alternate fasting, though this is one of the most common methods. On your eating days, you eat regular meals, while on the fasting day; your calorie consumption is reduced to 25 percent of the calories added during your eating day.

On fasting days, meals typically comprise starch, high fiber, sugar-free and good fat foods. Avoid artificially processed foods and fast food. Restrict your calorie consumption during non-fast days too. If weight loss is your main objective for practicing alternate fasting, keep your calorie intake below 1000 calories a day during non-fasting days, and 250 calories on alternate fasting days. Avoid giving in to the temptation of excessive indulgence during eating days.

For losing weight, you'll have to eat in moderation on all days. If you restrict your calorie intake on non-fasting days, you will eat less even on fasting days, thus helping you lose weight much quicker with intermittent fasting. Alternate fasting is known to be one of the best fasting methods from the view of reducing calorie consumption and losing weight. It may not be the best plan for people leading a more hectic life as switching between fasting and eating may not be suitable for people leading a hectic life.

The basis of alternate day fast is that you fast one day and consume regular meals the next day. This way instead of limiting or restricting what you want to eat all the time, you are only limiting your time for eating by half. On fasting days, you can consume unlimited amounts of calorie-free beverages such as water, unsweetened tea, and coffee. Those following a modified Alternate-day fasting plan can consume about 500 calories on their fasting days or meet about 20 to 25 percent of your body's energy needs. Dr. Krista Varady's "The Every-Other-Day Diet" is probably the most popular version of Alternate Fasting Plan.

This fasting type can offer weight loss benefits irrespective of whether you take the calories during lunch, breakfast, dinner or tiny meals spread across the day. According to research, people find it easier to fast on alternate days than adhere to the conventional daily calorie restriction for weight loss. Balance is the key here. While limiting your calorie intake on a daily basis, we often deprive our body of the opportunity to eat certain types of foods. This can quickly result in increased cravings, and subsequently giving up the diet plan to please our palate.

On the other hand, Alternate Fasting plan maintains a sort of balance. On certain days you resort to fasting while consuming regular meals on other days. A majority of studies use alternate-day fasting implemented in the modified version (500 calories a day on fasting days). This is known to be more sustainable than going on full fasts on certain fasting days. However, its efficiency remains the same.

Benefits of Alternate-Day Fasting

Alternate-day fasting is a type of intermittent fasting method where a person fasts for a day and can eat meals of their choice the following day. There are several versions of the alternate fasting plan, which also includes limiting calories on eating days. Research points to the fact that alternate-day fasting is a feasible dietary plan for protection against heart ailments (especially in adults suffering from obesity) and weight loss. Generally, on fasting days, a person can drink unlimited amounts of calorie-free drinks. Apart from this, they can consume around 20 to 25 percent of their everyday calorie needs (around 500 calories).

It can help in managing diabetes and cardiovascular ailments.

Research published in the British Journal of Diabetes and Vascular Disease has concluded that intermittent fasting aids in weight loss and enhances the body's cardiovascular mechanism. The same research also suggests that fasting can reduce instances of diabetes. Another research in 2014 indicates that alternate day fasts have the same advantages as that of a limited calorie diet, and can prevent heart diseases as well as diabetes.

It facilitates weight loss.

Alternate-day fasting has been closely linked with weight loss since for long now. Our bodies are wired to cope with starvation and the subsequent metabolic changes. When a person practices alternate-day fasting, the body's mechanism automatically ramps up. The result: our cells switch from using glucose as their main source of energy to using stored fat within the cells. Owing to this switch, triglycerides accumulated within the body are broken down and utilized as energy sources resulting in lower fat content within our body. Magic? Just plain simple science and the wonders of nature!

It helps in recovery of ailments such as cancer.

In a 2009 study, 10 patients suffering from different types of cancer were asked to go on an alternate-day fasting post their chemotherapy sessions. It was observed that fasting and chemotherapy were practical, safe and has the power to alleviate the effects of chemotherapy of the patient. Thus, alternate-day fasting can be beneficial for people recovering from ailments such as cancer.

It helps combat inflammation and oxidative stress.

According to research, when an overweight asthmatic person takes up alternate-day fasting, they are able to stick to the diet for a longer period than on a limited calorie diet. Apart from this, there are notable positive changes in the symptoms of the patient's pulmonary functions, owing to which he/she experiences lower oxidative stress and inflammation.

Extended Fasting

Extended fasting is known to be an extreme form of intermittent fasting. It is rage currently owing to its several documented benefits. While people usually fast for 16-20 hours during intermittent fasting, prolonged fasting is when the fasting goes beyond 48 hours (yes you read that right). Extended fasting is climbing popularity charts everywhere since it has started getting recognized as a way to increase your lifespan, reduce inflammation and prevent life-threatening ailments like cancer.

Benefits of Extended Fasting

Extended fasting is known to have several benefits with the most obvious one being weight loss. You'll tend to shed some pounds immediately for several reasons. First, your body is going to lose plenty of water. It will slowly deplete glycogen stored in the liver initially before moving on to the muscles. After these reserves are used, muscle glycogen is targeted. When your muscle glycogen is used, the process leads to a considerable loss of water. This is exactly why dieticians recommend consuming more salt and water during the ketosis phase. Once your body utilizes the available glycogen, it starts burning stored fat for meeting its energy requirements. This leads to the body getting into a metabolic ketosis state either by fasting or sticking to a ketogenic diet (nutritional ketosis).

Extended fasting can transform your body into a speedy fat burning mechanism. Since your body no longer possesses any dietary fat, it starts dipping into its own stored fat reserves. This is exactly why not eating for longer durations makes for an effective weight loss strategy. One of the things to keep in mind is to not make extended fasting your sole weight loss method in the long run. The reason – it may not be sustainable. You can use it in combination with other more "long haul" and sustainable weight loss methods. Prolonged fasting is not very sustainable as a long-term weight loss strategy though it can be used to meet short-term weight loss goals. Be assured though that if you do not have a more sustainable and long-term weight loss plan, all the weight that you lost through prolonged fasting is going to find its way to you all over again.

Another important benefit of extended fasting is autophagy or being in the fasting ketosis stage for an extended period. Autophagy translates to "self-eating" in Greek. As suggested by the term, when our body starts eating itself, we are in the autophagy stage. It can sound scary but it isn't as crazy as it sounds. The stage or process is all about recycling waste products from our body and taking care of oxidative stress. Autophagy has multiple anti-aging properties and is also known to facilitate muscular hypertrophy or growth. Prolonged fasting is being contemplated as a potential therapy for people suffering from cancer. There is plenty of research on how the effect of prolonged fasts in preventing certain types of cancers.

If you thought that was all, we aren't done yet. Extended fasts generally last between 48 to 120 hours, though fasters longer than this duration aren't completely unheard of. One of the most significant benefits of intermittent fasting is a considerable reduction of glycogen from the body.

An average human being can go without food for about 30 days. The number of days an individual can survive without food can varies from individual to individual. For example, a person with greater body fat can sustain longer than an active sportsperson with body fat amounting to 5-6 percent. This doesn't mean you should go on a month-long fast. It is not just unnecessary but downright unadvisable.

Extended fasting is also known to beneficial for the brain. Consider this – when food becomes scarce, you will need more of it for survival. This increases our critical thinking abilities, which helps us come up with strategic ways to look around for more food resources. Ketosis can be highly advantageous for the brain because it allows us to step outside our thought process comfort zones and look for more ways to meet the body's energy requirements. Extended fasting or even fasting, on the whole, is known to create a greater brain-derived neurotrophic factor for the human brain. This acts as a fertilizer for brand new neurons. Another benefit is that the brain synaptic plasticity increases and your resistance to stress does increase considerably.

Want to know more benefits or advantages of extended fasting? It is known for boosting your immune mechanism. Every time you fast for an extended period, your body's white blood cells reduce to cause an increase in the stem cell revival process. With the body's white blood cells depleted, it secretes an enzyme known as PKA that allows stem cells to rebuild and replenish the immune.

This is vital for people suffering from a spent immune system owing to harsh cancer treatments. Thus, fasting becomes a viable option to eliminate some side-effects of chemotherapy. This is exactly why you'll notice that people who practice regular fasting rarely get sick. Prolonged or extended fasting also releases adiponectin, which is a powerful anti-inflammatory agent that helps protect your body from chronic diseases.

Another important benefit of extended fasting is a boost in your willpower. A lot of people simply try fasting to test their willpower when it comes to abstaining from food. They want to check how much they can push themselves in the face of temptations. Prolonged fasting is a great way to test your discipline and willpower. It is also a wonderful way for expressing gratitude towards what you presently have. This mental discipline and willpower derived as a result of prolonged or extended fasting can be highly empowering. Getting too comfortable with or accustomed to something isn't a good idea. You should ideally get your body used to the feeling of discomfort once in a while so it learns to adapt itself well. This will lead to several health benefits.

Building a Nutritional Reserve While Fasting

This is applicable for any fast and not just prolonged fasting. One of the key features for determining the success of your fasting plan is "what to eat" to build your body's nutritional reserves for giving it something to fall back on during the fasting period. Several people practicing intermittent fasting, prolonged fasting and alternate fasting (which is also a type of intermittent fasting) focus on when you eat. There is an unnecessary obsession with eating and fasting at the right time. In a quest to stick to the right meal timings, what we eat often goes for a toss. It is all the more important to fill your body with nutrition if you are going to swing between the eating and fasting phase. In the absence of essential nutrients during the fasting phase, your body will invariably dip into available nutritive resources.

Here are some expert tips for building your body's nutritive reserves:

Drink lots of water – This is a no-brainer yet people never seem to understand it. They are always running low on energy and experiencing feelings of dehydration. If the fast demands completely avoiding the consumption of drinks and foods, ensure that you consume enough water before and after your meals. Avoiding water for long can cause dehydration, which comes with a fair share of ill effects.

Try and consume a nutrition-packed pre-fast meal – I am forever asked what foods one must consume before going on a fast. There really is no rule, though you should stick to high fibrous foods, whole grains, good fats, and protein-rich foods. Raw vegetables are also a good option. Avoid eating heavy and greasy meals before a fast. Keep it light, nutritious and healthy. Consume milk, nuts, cereals, and fruits before fasting. Remember, you are building a nutrition reserve for the body to dip into in the absence of fresh nutritional intake. Your body is going to rely on and function with the help of the nutrition resources you create before the fast.

Optimize nutrition during fasts – When you consume no food or less food, the nutritional value of what you eat is even more important to keep the body functioning normally. Avoid loading on fried foods and foods items high in sugar content. Baked vegetable preparations can be a good option. Similarly, fruits and light milk preparations (home-made) are good. This is of course for fasting where you are eating less food or limiting your calorie intake instead of completely going without food. Stay away from caffeinated drinks like aerated beverages, coffee, tea and so on as they can be diuretic and lead to a more rapid water loss owing to frequent urination.

Chapter Five: Fasting for Weight Loss – The Scientific Principle and How to Do It Right

Once we eat something, our body's blood sugar invariably increases. In combination with stored carbs, this forms the basis of our body's fundamental source of energy, which is burnt to fuel our day-to-day activities.

Let's understand that any form of fasting (if done right and in moderation) discussed in this book is not deprivation. It is more like spreading out the body's calorie intake from the conventional way of consuming three large meals a day. According to studies, the "three large meals and a few smaller snack meals" eating pattern is not compatible with the way our bodies have scientifically evolved.

Since prehistory, the food consumption pattern of humans was more random and erratic, heavily dependent on food availability. We didn't have access to "three large meals" and all the in-between trimmings available today. This is exactly why our bodies have adapted to going without food for a certain duration. We are not wired for eating frequently, which is completely opposite to what new-age dieticians and nutritionists recommend.

According to research, people following an intermittent fasting plan intake 10 to 15 percent lower calories on their non-fasting days in comparison to the fasting days. This means, their overall calorie intake is still lower than people who follow the conventional three large meals and snacks per day. When it comes to losing weight, calorie consumption is the most important component. Your calorie intake can be controlled when you eating windows reduce, and you eat healthier meals during the eating window. When you can't eat whenever you want or each time you experience hunger pangs, the body's total calorie intake can reduce.

Stored fat is burnt.

When you follow any form of fasting meal plan, the body's blood sugar level along with carbs dips. Hence, to sustain during the fasting phase, it has no option but to burn body fat for building energy to fuel the body's activities and function normally.

Fasting boosts HGH.

HGH is an incredible hormone that facilitates fat burning along with retaining muscle mass. This is important from the perspective of losing weight. Intermittent fasting has the ability to boost HGH by around 1,300 and 2,000 percent in women and men respectively according to research helmed by the Intermountain Medical Center.

One of the biggest advantages of fasting over other weight loss programs, diets, and meal plans is that the practitioner doesn't have to stress about losing muscle mass with weight. You can burn fat, while still retaining important muscle mass. This is something most weight loss plans find challenging to accomplish.

Lower overall calorie consumption.

This is a no-brainer. The lower your calorie intake, the more positive results your weighing scales will reveal. If you are searching for a fast an effective weight loss plan, the key is to limit calorie intake. You may experience cravings and hunger pangs during the initial fasting phases. However, over a period of time, the body adapts to going without food, while hunger pangs gradually subside. It comes to a stage, where you can go without food for long with feeling low on energy, weak or drained. By fasting over a period of time, you regularize the body's hunger hormone ghrelin, which facilitates appetite control.

When you fast, your body has lower insulin, and higher adrenaline as well as HGH. This facilitates the weight loss process.

Tips for Fast-Tracking Your Way to Weight Loss with Fasting

Fasting in combination with workouts can work wonders.

When our body's sugar, glycogen reserves, and insulin levels deplete, fat is burned for building energy. This happens irrespective of your physical activities or fitness regime. Now, just imagine the results you can get if you combine fasting with a regular fitness or physical activity regime.

The body's fat burning process with expedite, and you'll be able to burn fat much faster. Though high-intensity training or workouts are ideal, you can practice any form of physical fitness or activities such as running, dance, swimming, aerobics, cycling, and so on. Any form of regular and disciplined physical activity in combination with fasting can help speed up the weight loss process. Just ensure you are doing it right though. Don't do high-intensity workouts during your fasting window or immediately after breaking your fast. Maintain a balance between not wearing out your body during the fasting phase and ensuring overall physical fitness.

Stick to consuming low or zero calorie coffee an hour prior to your workout for more energy and additional fat burning in addition to the fat which is anyhow being burnt owing to intermittent fasting. Ensure you plan to fast during the 8-hour meal consuming window if you are following the 8-16 intermittent fasting method.

Typical fasting schedule for weight loss

Begin with a shorter fasting window and gradually work your way up by getting your body used to the concept of fasting. Ideally, start with an 8-10 fasting window (something that you are probably doing anyway now between dinner and breakfast the following day). Slowly, move it to 16-21 by skilling breakfast. The fasting window can be slowly increased by 30 to 60 minutes every week until you reach a fasting window your body is comfortable with depending on your weight loss objectives.

Avoid zooming from 8 hours to 16 hours straight in a one day. Once you are in the 16-hour fasting window, you are in an effective fat reduction stage.

Implementing a stress-free and effective fasting schedule

It is a nice practice to eat your dinner or final meal for the day at least 3-4 hours prior to sleeping. This ensures a majority of your fasting time is spent sleeping to avoid dealing with cravings and hunger pangs. Your body is positioned to get to work when it comes to burning fat for creating energy.

This is how a general intermittent fasting plan should look:

7:00 p.m. – Finish dinner

10:00 p.m. – Hit the bed

Following day

7:00 a.m. – Arise

7:00 a.m. to 11:30 a.m. – Go on with your everyday routine.

Now, you are probably only fasting for 4 waking hours, while the rest of the fasting window was spent sleeping. The three hours' post-dinner doesn't really count because you are already full after dinner.

11 a.m. -11:30 a.m. – Lunch post the 16-hour fasting period (hurray!!! Victory)

11 a.m. – 7 p.m. – You consume another meal or your dinner during this duration while also keeping your calorie intake in check.

7 p.m. – The fasting window starts again

Combating food cravings

One of the biggest challenges you'll deal with while fasting for weight loss is dealing with food cravings. The fact that you are sticking to low calorie and high fiber foods during your eating window makes these cravings even more compelling.

There will be cravings during the initial fasting stages. At times, it is perfectly alright to break the fast if you experience excessive dizziness, headaches, stomach ache or nausea. There can be other forms of discomfort too depending on your overall health and body composition. Avoid pushing it too hard. Keep going steadily until you accomplish 16 hours of fasting comfortably, which invariably happens when our body gets accustomed to going without food for extended periods.

Consume green tea, calorie-free coffee, warm water, and sparkling water for reducing hunger and food cravings. My favorite tip for curbing hunger during fasting is drinking a glass of warm water. If you are working, try consuming tea and coffee (calorie free) to keep you going during the fasting phase. Green tea is known to boost the body's metabolic rate, while also facilitating the fat burning process. This can help keep your hunger pangs in check. In a sense, if you do take in a tiny number of calories from the above-mentioned beverages, it is compensated for.

Eat whenever you feel like during the eating phase.

Most diets suggest when a person should eat, what they should eat and the total calorie intake they should stick to. If you are already on a diet plan that suggests the type of meals you should consume, you are probably keeping your total calorie intake below 1000 calories. This means as long as you do not exceed 1000 calories, you can eat whenever you like during the 8 (or whatever duration you are eating for) hour eating window. It can be phased out to a couple of meals comprising 500 calories each with a break of 4 hours in-between.

Control your carb, bad fat, and sugar intake.

If you are following a fasting plan such as intermittent fasting, you do not have a suggested list of what you must or must not eat. However, if you are following a fasting plan for the purpose of weight loss, you have to be mindful, conscious, and smart about your food choices.

The meals during your eating phase should comprise balanced, regular, and healthy meals. Avoid overeating to compensate for the fasting phase. One tip for eating less and still feeling full is to chew each morsel at least 20 times. This will help you eat more intentionally and mindfully.

Eliminate items such as bad fats, processed carbs, and sugar from your meals. Though fasting methods such as intermittent fasting are less rigid, combine your plan with eating right and exercising for optimal weight loss. Give white bread and white rice (also pasta) a miss, and instead opt for raw foods, high fiber, good fats, protein-rich and fresh foods. You'll soon begin to notice the difference in the way you look and feel.

Chapter Six: Unlocking the Secrets of Autophagy and Ketosis

Autophagy in Greek translates into self-eating. It is a normal physiological process in which the human body copes with the destruction of cells within the body. Autophagy is an intracellular degradation mechanism where the body's unwanted substances—such as damaged organelles, unwanted proteins, and pathogen agents—are digested. Later, the macromolecular bodies digested are released into the cytosol. Originally explained by Christian de Duve in 1963, autophagy comprises the sequestration of organelles along with cytoplasmic material into double-membrane vesicles known as autophagosomes and their delivery into the lysosomes for the lysosomal hydrolases' degradation.

This allows the process of autophagy to regulate the balance of protein composition within a cell to prevent a build-up of toxic waste or maintaining cellular organelle functions, eliminating invasive pathogens and helping sustain cells during prolonged starvation periods. The scientific relevance of autophagy was brought to light when the 2016 Nobel Prize in Physiology was awarded to Yoshinori Ohsumi for his autophagy mechanism discoveries.

Primarily, autophagy is the creation of a garbage bag that collects cellular material and then drops them near the cell's recycling center to be broken into various parts that can subsequently be recycled into brand new components.

Move over juice cleanses and new-age detox diets. Autophagy is the new buzz related to flushing toxins from the body, weight loss, anti-aging, and cleansing. Our cells make several membranes that are forever hunting for dead scraps and heavily worn cells. It gobbles up these cells, strips them for different parts, and the resultant molecules for sources of energy to fuel new cell parts. This is our body's primary recycling program that destroys the old to make way for the new. Think of autophagy as a process that allows us to become more efficient mechanisms to get rid of the old and make way for the new.

Benefits of Autophagy

Now that we understand this slightly complicated physiological process of autophagy, let's quickly run through its benefits.

1. It can increase your lifespan.

Throughout history, people's lifespans have increased despite unhealthy fad diets, crazy work schedules, and stressful lifestyles. Isn't it funny how humans have survived all the rigmarole and still manage to increase their lifespan over a period of time? This can be attributed to the tiny changes and transformations we have made over a period of time. Research has closely linked these changes to a protein that helps activate autophagy.

Does autophagy really expedite the process of living longer? There is no straightforward answer to this. For now, it may be safe to say that it is known to have disease-fighting properties that can give us a longer lifespan.

2. It promotes natural detoxification.

By cleaning out our body's damaged cells and proteins, autophagy facilitates a natural detox (move over exotic Alpine spas). It also lowers inflammation and helps you maintain glowing health. If you experience a feeling of tiredness and exhaustion, autophagy can come to your rescue. This is owing to the radicals that collect in your body's tissues and organs where they can lead to cell damage, while also disrupting regular processes. Triggering autophagy is one of the best ways to eliminate all substances from the body that are unwanted or holding you down. This is spring cleaning for the body at its best.

3. Slows the process of aging.

Studies reveal that inducing autophagy helps in slowing down the body's aging process. It has also been proven that it is known to delay neurodegenerative diseases such as Alzheimer's and Parkinson's disease. A study mentions how caloric reduction triggers autophagy, which is known to be the most powerful anti-aging discovery ever known to mankind. The process can be utilized to the fullest to keep your skin looking healthy, younger and glowing. It can also be used for fighting a number of skin conditions such as systematic lupus, skin infections, psoriasis, and vitiligo.

5 Ways to Eat Yourself or Induce Autophagy

No, it isn't as scary as I've made it sound here. It is pretty simple actually. To begin with, understand that autophagy is your body's response to stress. You are actually activating the body's stress mechanism to create some additional auto-cannibalism. As is the case, short-term discomfort brings plenty of long-term benefits. Here are three fundamentals techniques for boosting your autophagy

1. Exercise

If sweating, post-workout exhilaration, and grunting don't get you feeling all good, here's something to remember. Exercise induces stress on your body. Working out can play havoc with your muscles while causing small microscopic tears that your body rushes in full speed to heal. This makes you boost your muscle strength and resistance, thus reducing any further damage. Regular exercise and workouts are a popular way to unintentionally assist the body during the cleansing process. This means there really is something to the wonderful, rejuvenated, and fresh feeling you experience after a satisfying workout. Sticking to a regular and disciplined exercise schedule is one of the most widespread ways through which people help cleanse their own body although unintentionally.

One research viewed autophagosomes (structures created around the cell pieces that the body attempts to recycle). So what level of exercise is needed to create the autophagy phase? The answer isn't known yet. Exercise and a regular fitness routine have tons of benefits and are good overall for triggering some amount of autophagy. Tough workouts are even more sought after. You can practice some form of considerably intense exercise for optimal results. One doesn't really have to go running on the treadmill for 45 minutes to an hour to stimulate autophagy. Any regular high-intensity training that pumps up your heart rate and goes on for 25-30 minutes per day should be good enough.

2. Reducing carb intake

Unless you are living in a rabbit hole, you've heard of ketosis. It is one of the most popular diets among everyone from bodybuilders to people looking to increase their lifespan. The objective is to decrease your carb intake to such a reduced level that the body doesn't have any option but to convert fat into an energy source. Ketosis is the ultimate autophagy hack. You experience plenty of metabolic advantages and transformations of fasting without fasting. Ketosis assists in reducing body fat while still retaining muscle. Some research suggests that it helps our body combat cancerous tumors and reduces the propensity of diabetes. Ketosis is also known to fight certain brain disorders such as epilepsy.

Keto diets are typically high fat. In these diets, about 60 and 70 percent of a person's overall calories originate from fat. Then again, the protein comprises about 20 to 30 percent calories, while carbs stay at 50 grams a day. Little wonder then that researchers are working to include all benefits of autophagy in a single pill, though it's still a long way off. Inducing autophagy through chemicals would probably be simpler than fasting or dieting but researchers still have a long way to go before they accomplish it.

3. Fasting

This is the reason autophagy finds itself mentioned in this book. Fasting is one of the most powerful ways to induce autophagy, which is known to have plenty of benefits. How does the act of skipping meals invoke autophagy? It is simple! Skipping meals is stressful for the body. The body doesn't take to it instantly. However, there are plenty of benefits in the long run. Like we've discussed above, several studies have collaborated the fact that occasional fasting has plenty of benefits such as reduced risk of diabetes and heart ailments (which can also be owing to autophagy). It is amazing how research has emphasized specifically on the manner in which fasting facilitates autophagy within the human brain, suggesting that it could probably one of the most powerful ways to reduce neurodegenerative diseases such as Parkinson's and Alzheimer's.

In a research (published on Scientific American), intermittent fasting was also proven to enhance our cognitive functions, neuroplasticity and brain structure, which facilitates easier learning for the brain. However, since the study was conducted on rodents, it wasn't conclusive enough to establish anything. During intermittent fasting, practitioner generally goes without food from 12 to 36 hours at a stretch, ensuring your body gets a lot of water. This period of fasting can also be combined with light exercises such as stretching and yoga for increasing your chances of triggering autophagy.

4. Protein fast

You can enjoy the advantages of autophagy by undertaking a protein fast, where your protein consumption is restricted to 25 grams a day. The objective behind a protein fast is to offer your body an entire day to recycle old proteins that can lead to inflammation if accumulated for long. You can cleanse your cells without causing muscle loss, which helps you stay lean. According to research, when we restrict our protein intake, it compels the body to consume its own proteins and unwanted toxins that have been accumulated. This lowers the amount of protein lingering around. Some studies (nicbi.nlm.nih.gov) reveal that protein deficiency helps create autophagy since it works closely with fasting. Being protein deficient reduces the body's insulin levels along with mTOR (mechanistic Target of Rapamycin) levels, which regulate cell growth and the body's metabolism rate.

When the mTOR level plunges and then builds back, it assists in rebuilding and repairing our cells so we can build leaner muscle. It is also known to have plenty of other benefits such as controlling the process of aging along with major disorders such as diabetes and cancer. Keep in mind that you do not have to restrict your protein intake on a daily basis. Protein deficiency over a period of time has more disadvantages than advantages. You can go on a protein fast over a 24-hour period once or twice a week (think the 5:2 intermittent fasting method). A natural way to go on a protein fast is following the ketogenic diet.

5. Ketogenic diet

Several people discover, much to their delight, that the fastest and best way to induce autophagy is by following the ketogenic diet along with a reduction in the body's protein intake. The scientific principle behind this is that proteins can be converted into sugar when you consume them in excess amounts.

Fat, on the contrary, is unable to do this. When you adopt a high-fat, low carb and low-protein diet plan, it switches your source of energy to ketones and mimics a natural fasting. To cut a long story short, you can induce autophagy simply by staying in the ketosis stage.

Apart from this, by decreasing your body's protein and carb consumption, you'll be limiting the number of toxins making their way into your body. Thus, there will be fewer toxins for the body to flush out, which helps autophagy show its full strength. Therefore, people adopting a Keto diet experience a feeling of renewal and rejuvenation. It has to do with fewer toxins and a healthy overall makeover.

Ketosis

You'll probably come across the term ketosis when you look up matter on weight loss. Let's understand what it is in the first place before moving on to how you can activate it and use it to fast track your weight loss goals.

Ketosis is a regular metabolic process undertaken by your body to keep functioning normally. When the body doesn't derive sufficient carbs from the food you consume to facilitate the cell burning process for energy, fat is burnt in its place. During this phase, ketones are made in the body. Ketones are nothing but acids that build up in our blood and are discharged from the body through urine. In tiny amounts, they are an indication that our body is breaking down fat. However, high ketone levels can be poisonous and fatal for the body and lead to a condition called ketoacidosis.

When we consume healthy, balanced and nutritious meals, our body regulates the amount of fat that is burnt, and ketones aren't made or utilized as such. However, when you cut back on calories and carbs, the body automatically switches to ketosis for meeting its energy needs. This process can also occur after exercising for long periods of time. In people suffering from uncontrolled diabetes, ketosis signals non-usage of sufficient insulin.

Ketosis is risky when ketones keep building up. A high ketone build-up can cause dehydration and a disturbance in the brain's chemical balance. Predictably, ketosis is a much sought-after weight loss technique. Low-carb meal plans include the initial part of both Paleo and Atkins diet, which emphasize protein intake for fueling the body. Apart from helping you burn fat, ketosis controls your hunger and helps maintain muscle.

In an average healthy non-pregnant person who doesn't suffer from ailments such as diabetes, ketosis normally occurs after 3-4 days of consuming lower than 50 grams of carbs a day. Ketosis can also be activated by fasting.

There have been some studies indicating that ketogenic diets can lower the risk of heart ailments. Still, other research suggests that it can also help with those with type 2 diabetes, metabolic syndrome, and insulin resistance. There is on-going research about the effects of a ketogenic diet on cancer, nervous system disorders, acne, and polycystic ovary syndrome.

Here are some quick facts on ketosis that will help you understand the state even more effectively:

- Ketosis happens when the body doesn't have enough access to its fundamental fuel source – glucose.

- Ketosis is a physiological condition where our body's fat reserves are broken down for generating energy (an acid called ketones is also developed during the process) in the absence of glucose.

- It is important to note that pent-up ketone levels can be dangerous. When your body's ketone levels rise, the blood's acidity also soars, leading to a high-risk condition called ketoacidosis.

- A ketogenic diet is often followed by people who intend to lose weight by compelling the body to break down and burn its stored fat resources for energy.

- People suffering from type 1 diabetes are likelier to develop the fatal ketoacidosis condition, which requires immediate medical treatment to prevent diabetic coma.

Can Ketosis Be Beneficial?

Ketosis may have a positive impact on cardiovascular ailments, metabolic syndrome, and diabetes. It may also help enhance boost HDL cholesterol levels (also referred to as good cholesterol). However, on the whole, these health benefits can be more connected with losing excess weight and consuming healthier meals than simply reducing the intake of carbs.

The ketogenic diet has been employed under medical supervision to lower seizures in epilepsy struck children who fail to respond to other treatment forms. Research has suggested ketogenic diet can also benefit adults suffering from epilepsy, although more studies are needed to collaborate this finding.

Ketosis is known to boost our memory, boost cognitive functions, facilitate better clarity of thought, and lead to seizure control. It is also believed to reduce migraines. Researchers have discovered a close link between a ketogenic diet and an increase in cognitive functions plus memory power (Neurobiology of Aging 2004 Mar 25 (3): 311-4) in adults who formerly struggled with it. There is growing research that suggests improvement at multiple stages of dementia. Ketosis is also observed to be effective in fighting Parkinson's disease.

In general, ketosis is believed to be beneficial for mental clarity, focus, reducing migraine intensity, and improving the brain's chemical balance for boosting cognitive functions and memory.

According to a study published in Dom D'Agostino's lab, it was observed that ketone supplementation reduces tumor visibility and increases survival of mice struck with metastatic cancer.

Ketosis is also known to increase energy levels and sleep. During the fourth or fifth day of being on a ketogenic diet, a majority of people have observed an increase in their overall energy levels in addition to reduced carb cravings. Reason – regulated insulin levels and an easily available energy source. Research has revealed that ketogenic dieting enhances your sleep by reducing REM and boosting slow-wave sleeping patterns. While the exact cause for this still remains unknown, it can most likely be attributed to the complicated biochemical shift in the brain's utilization of ketones (as fuel for generating energy) in combination with other body tissues that burn fat directly.

Ketosis is also known to reduce inflammation, thus fighting conditions such as psoriasis, arthritis, IBS, eczema, and acne. One of the widely known benefits of ketogenic dieting is anti-inflammation, which helps those following the diet fight a series of health problems associated with inflammation. Studies have shown that the fundamental player responsible for several inflammatory ailments is subjugated by BHS, which is one of the key ketones generated by following a ketogenic diet. Thus, ketosis has a significantly positive effect on conditions such as acne, eczema, arthritis, psoriasis, and other inflammation-related ailments.

Muscle gain and endurance is another noted benefit of following a ketogenic diet or reaching ketosis. BHB is known to facilitate muscle gain. There have been several accounts of bodybuilders employing the ketogenic technique for gaining muscle and reducing fat.

Ketosis is critical in preventing heart diseases, lowering blood pressure, reducing triglycerides and regulating cholesterol profiles. These are again a direct result of keeping the body's blood glucose levels low and regulated. A ketogenic diet can facilitate the process of controlling blood pressure and reducing triglyceride levels.

While you may be baffled by how consuming higher fat percentage can reduce triglycerides, the truth is that the intake of excess like fructose is the key to boosting triglycerides. The body's HDL and LDL particles, which is utilized by moving cholesterol and fat, are also positively impacted by a ketogenic diet. It facilitates an increase in HDL or good cholesterol and improves the LDL or bad cholesterol profile.

Getting into the Ketosis Stage

Like we discussed above, ketosis is a regular metabolic process of the body that is known to offer multiple health benefits. During the process of ketosis, our body converts stored fat into ketones and starts utilizing them for meeting its energy requirements.

There has been significant research linking diets that cause ketosis to weight loss and other health benefits. Owing to the appetite-suppressing feature, ketosis is known to be an effective weight loss approach. Upcoming research has also suggested that ketosis may be effective against several neurological disorders along with type 2 diabetes and other conditions. This brings us to the main point now—how does one get into the ketosis state?

Accomplishing the state of ketosis is not an easy process. It takes some planning, detailing and work. While some people mistakenly believe that it is as simple as cutting your carb intake, there's more to achieving a state of ketosis.

Here are some of the most effective tips to help you get into the ketosis state:

1. Reduce carb intake – This is probably the most important pointer for getting into the ketosis state. In normal conditions, your body's cells utilize sugar or glucose as the primary source of energy for fueling the body's day to day activities. However, a majority of your body's cells also utilize other energy sources, which include ketones. Glucose is stored in our muscles and liver in the form glycogen. When we reduce our carb intake, these liver and muscle-stored glycogen reserves start depleting, which directly results in a hormone insulin reduction. This, in turn, leads to the release of fatty

acids from the body's stored fat reserves. Our liver performs the function of converting these fatty acids into beta-hydroxybutyrate, ketone bodies acetone and acetoacetate. Ketones are employed as energy sources to fuel certain brain functions.

There is no universally stipulated carb restriction level for inducing the ketosis state. It varies from person to person. While some people require to restrict their net carb consumption (the sum total of carbs minus fiber) to 20 grams a day, others can accomplish ketosis while consuming double of this carb quantity. It all boils down to your body type, physiological functions, and overall health. It is precisely for this reason that diets such as the widely popular Atkins diet suggest that your carb intake should be limited to 20 or lesser grams a day to guarantee to accomplish the ketosis state.

Once you achieve this state, you can keep including small quantities of carbs in your diet slowly. Ensure that the process of ketosis is not disturbed by your carb intake. The idea is to add small amounts gradually, while still maintaining ketosis. If you intend to accomplish the ketosis state for therapeutic purposes, it should be implemented only under the advice and supervision of a doctor. Restricting your calorie consumption to 20-25 net grams a day reduced blood sugar as well as insulin levels, thus triggering the release of fatty acid reserves that are converted into ketones by the liver.

2. Step up your physical activity – An increasing number of studies suggest that staying in the ketosis stage can have a positive impact of some forms of athletic training such as endurance. Increasing your physical activity and sticking to a regular fitness regime can help you accomplish ketosis.

How does this happen? When we exercise or perform intense physical activities, our body's glycogen reserves deplete. In normal circumstances, these depleted reserves are replenished when we consume carbs, which are then broken into glucose and finally, glycogen. However, when our carb intake is restricted, glycogen reserves stay low. The liver then steps up its generation of ketones that can be utilized as an alternate fuel for muscles in the absence of regular energy sources. Research has indicated that when ketone concentrations in our blood are low, exercise boosts the speed with which ketones are generated. However, when there is a high concentration of ketones in the blood, the ketones actually reduce for a shorter duration with exercise. Thus, exercise may not produce any negative results irrespective of your blood ketone proportion.

Apart from this, research suggests that working out during the fasting state increases the body's ketone levels. It is important to know that though exercise boosts ketone production, it takes roughly 7-28 days for our body to get accustomed to utilizing fatty acids and ketones as main energy sources. You won't skyrocket your way into ketosis by exercising in a fasted state for a day or two. It will take time, patience, observation and effort to reach there.

On the whole, stepping up your physical activity can boost our body's ketone levels when you are on a restricted carb diet. This effect can also be increased by working out while fasting.

3. Increase good fat intake – Including healthier fat foods in your diet can increase your ketone levels and help you accomplish ketosis. A low-carb ketogenic diet not just reduces your carb intake but is also high in good fat. Ketogenic diets followed for weight loss, boosting athletic performance, and improving metabolic health generally offer 60 to 80 percent of calories only from fat. The original ketogenic diet that was utilized for epilepsy has an even higher concentration of fat (generally 90 percent of its calories are provided through fat).

High fat consumption doesn't necessarily mean increased ketone levels so don't make that the basis of your diet plan. Since fat comprises a sizeable percentage of your ketogenic diet plan, it is vital to pick high-quality sources of good fat to make your diet effective. Some major sources of good fats include coconut oil, olive oil, tallow, butter, and avocado oil. Apart from this, there are several nutritious high-fat foods which feature low carb content. If you want to get into ketosis for losing weight, it is vital to ensure that you are not increasing your total calorie count as it may not offer the desired results.

4. Go on a short fast - Another method for reaching ketosis is by going without food for several hours. Several people accomplish a mild ketosis stage from dinner to breakfast, when you go without food for a good 10-12 hours. Children suffering from epilepsy are sometimes subjected to a 24-48 hour fast under medical supervision before they are put on a ketogenic diet. This is done to accomplish the ketosis state faster for controlling seizures. Intermittent fasting, which involves going on frequent short duration fasts, is also known to be effective for inducing ketosis.

Fat fasting is another approach that produces results similar to fasting while also boosting ketones. When fasting on fats, a person consumes around 1,000 calories a day, 80 to 90 percent of which are derived from fat. Thus, low caloric intake combined with high fat can help you get into ketosis faster.

Since a fat fast has low protein and caloric content, it should not be implemented for more than four to five days to avoid excess muscle mass loss. It can be challenging to follow a fat fast for more than a couple of days. Fasting such intermittent fasting as well as fat fast facilitate the process of accomplishing ketosis.

5. Maintain sufficient protein intake – Accomplishing the state of ketosis needs protein consumption that is sufficient, though not excessive. The original ketogenic diet utilized for epilepsy is limits both carb and protein intake for optimizing ketone levels. Some research suggests that the same diet can also be advantageous for cancer patients as it inhibits tumor growth. For a majority of people though restricting protein for boosting production of ketones isn't known to be healthy.

To begin with, your body needs sufficient protein for supplying amino acids to the liver, which are then utilized for gluconeogenesis, which literally means "building new glucose." During this process, our liver becomes a source of glucose for some parts of the brain and kidney along red blood cells that are unable to utilize ketones as an energy source. Also, your protein intake should be enough to maintain muscle mass when the body's carb intake is restricted especially when you are reaching ketosis for weight loss. Losing weight can generally result in the loss of fat as well as muscle. Consuming enough protein on an extremely low-carb ketogenic plan can lead to the preservation of muscle mass. Multiple studies have revealed that preserving muscle mass and performance of physical activities is optimized when our protein intake stays between 0.55 to 0.77 grams for a pound of lean mass. In weight loss research, extremely low carb plans with sufficient protein intake (within the range specified above) have been shown to not just induce but also maintain ketosis.

The bottom line is consuming very little protein can cause loss of vital muscle mass, while excess protein intake can inhibit the process of ketone production.

6. Evaluate ketone levels and adjust your diet accordingly – Pretty much like everything in diet plans, nutrition, and weight loss programs, accomplishing and maintain ketosis doesn't have universal rules. It is a more individualized process. Something that suits someone else may not suit you. Similarly, you may find some tips working more effectively for you than another person. Keep testing your body's ketone levels to ascertain you're on track when it comes to meeting your ketosis goals.

There are three fundamental types of ketones (acetoacetate, acetone, and beta-hydroxybutyrate) that are measured through a person's urine, breath, and blood. Acetone is spotted in the breath, and research has concluded that measuring acetone breath levels is a fairly dependable way to examine ketosis in ketogenic diet followers. A "ketonix" meter is utilized for measuring the breath's acetone levels. You breathe into the meter and watch out for a color flash indicating whether you are currently in ketosis as well as your ketosis level. Another way to measure ketones is using a blood ketone meter. It functions as a glucose meter. A strip with a tiny blood drop is put into the meter to measure your blood's beta-hydroxybutyrate levels. It is also a valid indicator of your body's ketosis levels.

Ketones in urine known acetoacetate can be measured with the help of ketone urine stripes. These strips are dipped into the ketosis practitioner's urine and depending on the shade the strip turns into (different shades of purple and pink), the person's ketone level can be determined. According to a recent study, our ketones are at their highest level during the early hours of the day and post-dinner while following the ketogenic diet plan. Using any of the methods mentioned above, you can measure your body ketone levels and make the necessary changes to your diet based on your individualized health condition, goals and comfort levels. Measuring ketones is a good way to gauge if you need to make any changes for accomplishing ketosis.

Chapter Seven: Fasting Myths Debunked

We've all heard information about how fasting can be bad or plain unhealthy. However, let me state upfront—a majority of junk you've heard about fasting doesn't have any scientific basis. Here's debunking the most common fasting myths you've heard.

Myth 1 – Fasting slows down the body's metabolism.

Metabolism is the body's energy fuel for keeping your cells functioning normally. It is an aggregation of all the physiological functions occurring in your body to keep you alive. For a majority of the time, your base metabolic rate is closely linked to your weight.

The origins of this myth are unknown, and it is plain false. Despite the widespread belief that our metabolism slows down with fasting, studies have suggested that the only thing that matters is the total amount of food you take and the not the pattern of consuming this food. This is to suggest that the frequency in which you eat or your meal timings don't determine the body's composition. Even during fasts like intermittent or alternate-day fasting, the reason for eating and fasting at specific timings is to consume less food overall, and not burn the body's existing fat for energy. It isn't so much about when you eat.

The most important consideration is the amount of food you eat with regards to body composition and weight. It also depends a lot of the quality of the food you eat. Your body's metabolism is a sum total of everything that is required to survive. It isn't some mysterious gut fire! You don't have to obsess over ramping it up constantly. Rather, attempt to optimize it in a healthy and balanced way.

Fasting doesn't lower your metabolism, nor is it the same as starvation, contrary to popular misconception. The very concept of starvation is a major fasting myth—unless a person is actually starving by choice. Fasting and starving aren't the same. Factually, you are burning the number of calories your body is slated to burn. Other than adding exercise, there isn't a way to shed more calories. Through fasting, there are only a stipulated number of calories your body is geared to burn. Therefore, the only way to lose weight through fasting is to consume less food or exercise or do both.

To say that eating enhances your body's metabolism is like saying that keeping your ears open all the time improves health: it is a statement without meaning. On the contrary, fasting offers your digestive mechanism an opportunity to rest. Pretty much like blinking offers respite to our eyes.

Ever wondered why people who consume meals every few hours still manage to shed weight? Frequent diets are effective as long as they operate within the principle of calorie deficit. The real issue arises when over a period of time frequent eating causes reduced insulin sensitivity and other health issues.

Myth 2 – You'll gain weight once you stop fasting.

If you are fasting to knock off a few extra pounds and appear all svelte, well-toned, and fit, you'll have plenty of naysayers discouraging you from going on a fast by stating that it is pointless or all the weight you lose will pile back on again once you stop fasting. They couldn't be more wrong.

If your main objective for fasting is weight loss, you were probably taking in more calories than you were shedding. Most likely, you wanted to reverse the process for accomplishing your weight loss goals. When you stop fasting and revert to former eating patterns, you'll obviously regain weight. The reason is simple—you are back to the initial process of taking in more calories than you were utilizing. What has this got to do with fasting? It is simply about the discipline and balance you maintain in your meal plans post fasting.

Just because you fasted, you can't go back to your old ways and miraculously expect not to pile on the pounds if you aren't eating right. If you are consuming unhealthy, greasy, and high-calorie meals, you will obviously put on weight; previous fasting will not help you avoid this. You know the definition of insanity, right? If you keep doing what you have always done, you will keep getting the same results. If you want something different, you must be prepared to do something that you've never done. If you expend more calories than you consume through balanced eating and exercise, you'll be able to maintain your post fasting results. It is as simple as that.

Long term fasting and weight loss results entail changes in your lifestyle. Are you prepared to make these changes? You have to create a series of new and long-term habits that become the basis of a balanced and healthy lifestyle. Don't see fasting as some all-in-one miraculous pill for your weight loss and health goals. If anything, it can help you meet your short-term weight loss or health goals. It won't help you sustain results in the long run if you get back to unhealthy food and lifestyle habits.

Change is brought about by thinking, acting and eating differently, along with creating a mechanism for sustaining this change. One of the most widespread misconceptions about this myth is that a person gains weight instantly after the fast stops. This will happen only if you end up overeating and overcompensating for the reduced calorie intake during your fasting phase. If you end up eating much more than usual after the fast in a bid to overcompensate or consume extra calories, it's a no-brainer you will pack on extra pounds.

I've heard some people confidently say that weight loss during fasting is merely a reduction in water weight and muscle glycogen. This may be partly true. However, there's much more to it. The reality is that a fast practitioner will shed body fat in some form. It may not be a speedy or immediate process. However, if you stick to the fasting rules in a disciplined and determined manner over a period of time, you'll definitely see results.

Fat loss is not an instant process, it is gradual. Water weight, on the contrary, can be quickly shed. Therefore, fasting isn't really about reducing water weight.

Myth 3 – Fasting keeps you low on energy.

Here's another fasting bubble to burst. Yes, during the initial days of your fasting you may experience a feeling of dizziness or of being low on energy. This is especially true for people whose bodies are accustomed to fasting or who are habituated to eating every couple of hours. The body will go into some form of shock or take time to get accustomed to going without food. However, once your body adapts to a fasting lifestyle, there'll be no looking back. You will not feel low on energy by skipping meals or limiting your calorie intake. On the contrary, you'll end up feeling much lighter, more energetic, and generally positive. Seasoned fast practitioners are always vibrant, positive, and vigorous. They have no dearth of energy!

Think of it like this—hunger can be the most basic motivator that drives us. Why do predators go on a hunting spree in the most extreme conditions when they are hungry? When we experience hunger pangs, we've spent a majority of our energy. There is almost nothing left to fall back on. When you are hungry during a fast, your body is all geared up for getting the toughest job done.

The way to deal with this is not to concentrate on the hunger. Shift your focus elsewhere instead of thinking about when you are going to eat your next meal. Stay busy and distracted. While some people say (and even I have mentioned this) that one shouldn't fast on very stressful and physically taxing days, you can fast on days when you know you will be busy just to shift focus away from the hunger. Fasting can be a highly pleasant, fulfilling, and manageable experience if you are equipped with the right coping mechanism.

Some smart self-confessed dieticians will advise eating small meals periodically to keep your hunger in check. According to a recent study **(https://www.ncbi.nlm.nih.gov/pubmed/20339363)**, three high protein meals a day leads to a greater feeling of satiation and appetite/hunger control than six high protein meals. Of course, eating frequently works for some people and it depends entirely on the eating pattern your body is comfortable with. However, absolute statements such as "eating frequently curbs hunger" aren't true. In fact, there are no absolutes when it comes to determining how many meals should be consumed in a day. It depends on your body's requirements and unique composition. These myths often originate from lab studies that have little relevance with real-world eating patterns. Present research reveals that a balanced and normal diet with protein intakes that are generally followed in regular, nonrestricted diets indicate greater appetite control when consuming fewer and bigger meals than smaller and more frequent meals.

Myth 4 – Eating smaller meals keeps your blood sugar level in check.

According to diet experts, eating small meals frequently helps you keep your hunger in check while still fueling your energy levels.

There is an inherent psychological fear (yes, I call it psychological rather than physiological) associated with not eating often. We think we will suffer from hunger (conditioned as we are to equate frequent eating with a sound mind and body) and cognitive impairment if we don't eat often. Logically, consider the evolutionary effects of this notion for a while. If this were true, man has always been fasting either intentionally or unintentionally throughout history. There have been natural calamities such as famines and floods that have compelled people to fast. Do you really think we would be surviving or functioning normally if eating frequently was critical to our existence? The truth is, it isn't necessary.

Overhyped food companies peddling their unhealthy products will have you believe that eating frequently is integral to good health. This is nothing but marketing manipulation at the highest level, tricking you into believing that you have to keep eating frequently to survive.

Honestly, regulating blood sugar level isn't a top priority. Our body has developed several effective pathways to ensure that it will happen during the most extreme conditions. It will take around 84 fasting hours to reach a state where your blood sugar level has plunged enough to have detrimental consequences on the mental state. There's no way a few hours of fasting can cause you a mental misbalance—unless you are suffering from a medical condition.

Even post 84 hours of fasting, the affected mental state is a temporary process when the brain adapts to the utilization of ketones. While fasting for 48 hours or during extreme calorie deprivation, the body's blood sugar stays within a normal range. Our mental performance isn't negatively affected by it.

Blood sugar is one of the many short-haul feedback components used for regulating hunger. The widespread notion that reduced blood sugar leads to hunger is misplaced and incorrect. Low blood sugar doesn't automatically translate into hunger, and shouldn't sound your alarm bells. Low sugar is merely an indication of a lower range or threshold. This can be subject to multiple factors like a habitual diet, genetics, and the body's energy intake. Most significantly, it relies on entrenched meal plans, controlled by ghrelin and other hormones. Primarily, this translates into blood sugar changes following a meal pattern we are used to. The notion that a plunge in blood sugar results in hunger doesn't really have a clear basis. It is an attempt to explain why some people are easily able to cope with regular fasting periods without any negative side-effects.

Myth 5: Fasting causes muscle loss.

This myth probably originates from the notion that it is vital to have a steady intake of amino acids into the body to prevent muscle loss. Our bodies absorb protein at an extremely slow rate. After a massive, high-protein meal, amino acids make their way into our bloodstream for many hours.

Protein catabolism poses a challenge only during periods of extended fasting. This occurs when the body's stored glycogen starts depleting. To maintain blood glucose, the amino acid is converted into glucose. This happens slowly, and if amino acids cannot be obtained through food, protein is taken from the body's stored reserves such as muscles.

Myth 6: Skipping breakfast makes you fat.

Skipping breakfast is closely linked with increased weight according to popular perception. People who skip breakfast show a general disregard for health and healthy eating. Their eating may be more erratic or impulse driven, which is responsible for the weight gain. Again, nothing could be further from the truth. Weight gain doesn't really have to do with skipping breakfast as there is no scientific basis to this notion. Though there is no scientific basis to support the notion, people believe that skipping breakfast is closely linked with higher body weight. People who skip breakfast are likelier to diet, which means by default, there are higher chances of them being heavier than people who do not diet.

Bear in mind that those people who skip breakfast for no reason at all aren't the type who are mindful about leading a healthy lifestyle or understanding their body's nutritional needs. They are folks who probably eat in a more erratic manner or lead excessively busy lives.

They are the type of people who go on crash diets and eat on the rebound. All of this plays havoc with the body and brings all the weight right back.

At times, there is an argument to consume breakfast regularly since humans, in general, are more insulin sensitive in the early hours of the day. Yes, we become more insulin sensitive after fasting overnight or rather our insulin sensitivity is at its peak during the day's first meal. Insulin sensitivity reduces after the body's glycogen is spent. If you haven't eaten for about 9-10 hours, your liver glycogen slightly depletes. This increases insulin sensitivity, and it can happen at any time when you go without food for over 8 hours. It hasn't anything to do with special powers of the morning hour. So, there's nothing true about breakfast being the most important meal of the day or that skipping breakfast leading to weight loss. Insulin sensitivity occurs whenever you fast, whether overnight or during the day, since it has to do with the physiological process regarding the depletion of glycogen. This has no relevance to the time of the day or to the biological impact of time on the body.

Myth 7: Our brain needs a constant glucose supply.

Some people are of the view that if we don't consume carbs every few hours, our brains won't function effectively. This is rooted in the belief that our brain can only utilize glucose or blood sugar for meeting its energy requirements or fueling the body's normal functions. There is absolutely no truth to this. However, what is omitted from this discussion is that our body is capable of generating glucose through the process of gluconeogenesis. This won't even be required in most cases of fasting since our body has enough stored glucose reserves within which can be used to fuel the brain for many hours. Even during long-term fasts, low carb diets, and starvation, our bodies are accustomed to generating ketones from dietary fat. Ketone bodies can offer energy to the brain for lowering its glucose needs significantly.

During a prolonged fast, our brain can effortlessly sustain itself with the help of ketone bodies in addition to glucose generated from fats and proteins. If our brains truly needed a constant glucose supply, it would make sense from an evolutionary point of view that we shouldn't be able to sustain without a perpetual source of carbohydrates. However, this is a fallacy. If this was the case, humans as a race would've become extinct thousands of years ago. Primitive man didn't have access to a regular supply of carbs. Some people report that they undergo a hypoglycemic feeling when they stop eating for some time. If you find that this feeling is something you experience, you may want to go with a higher frequency meal plan after consulting a medical practitioner.

The bottom line is that our body is capable of generating glucose to fuel the brain with its required quota of energy—even when you are in a long-term fasting phase or starvation. Some parts can also utilize ketone bodies for energy.

Conclusion

I genuinely hope the book was able to help you gain invaluable and little-known insights into the process of fasting, its benefits, the most advantageous and suitable fasting methods, and how to avoid the pitfalls or dangers of fasting.

The next step is to stop *merely* dreaming about stunning results and to take action immediately. If you are healthy and have no medical issues, special health requirements, or conditions, there is really no ideal time to fast—the right time is when you decide to do it.

I've added lots of little-known techniques, tried-and-tested strategies, and actionable pointers/guidelines for helping you begin your journey on the road to healthy, mindful, and purposeful eating. From fasting beginners to seasoned dieters, anyone can enjoy the benefits of the easy-to-follow, straightforward, and effective fasting strategies mentioned in this book.

Select a fasting plan that best suits your lifestyle, weight loss goals, and general health objectives. No one plan is better than another.

The one that is appropriate for your goals and lifestyle is the best for you. Likewise, don't give up when it gets challenging. Take a break from fasting or eat a little before your fasting window ends—but don't quit.

Lastly, if you enjoyed reading the book, please take some time out to share your thoughts by posting a review on Amazon. It'd be greatly appreciated!

Here's to your purposeful eating, weight loss, and healthy living!

If you enjoyed this individual book on Water Fasting, a review on Amazon would be greatly appreciated because it helps me to create more books that people want.

Thanks for your support!

Part 2: Autophagy

Unlock the Secrets of Weight Loss, Anti-Aging, and Healing with Intermittent and Extended Water Fasting

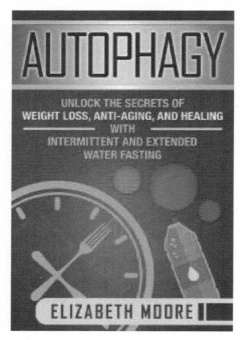

Introduction

The following chapters will discuss everything that you need to know about the process of autophagy and how it can improve your daily life. Without the process of autophagy working properly in your body, dead and damaged cells and proteins start to build up. These parts get there through normal wear and tear on the body, but they need to be reduced to keep your body healthy. If they aren't removed and are instead allowed to just sit around, they can cause inflammation, along with a whole bunch of other health conditions.

The autophagic process is needed to ensure that your body can clear out these damaged and dead parts of cells effectively and timely. When this process is allowed to do its work, it can help reduce inflammation in the body, can make room for new cells throughout, and can prevent many other diseases.

One of the best ways to induce this process is to go on a fast. Whether you choose to try out intermittent fasting and some of the shorter-term fasts that come with it or if you want to go all-out and try an extended fast, you will find that fasting can put you into the autophagic process and get you the results, along with many others, that you are looking for. We will discuss how fasting can work with autophagy and why it is such a good idea.

For some people, fasting may not be the best choice. Due to medical and health conditions, they may not want to put themselves at risk through fasting. The good news is that there are other methods that you can choose, such as a protein fast, the ketogenic diet, and exercise, that will help you to get the same results without having to go for long periods without eating.

This guidebook details all of these topics and more. We will talk more about the benefits of autophagy, how to do a good fasting period to induce autophagy, the results that others have been able to get from this process, and even some tips that make fasting easier to start on and stick with in the long run. There is so much to learn about and understand when it comes to the autophagic process – and this guidebook aims to help with it all.

When you are ready to improve your health, reduce your risks of inflammation and other diseases, fight off cancer, and even lose weight, then make sure to check out this guidebook and learn more about the autophagic process.

Chapter 1: The What and the Why – What Really Is Autophagy, and Why Are People Interested in It?

Even if your body is healthy and you aren't suffering from any illnesses, diseases, or pain, cells are constantly being damaged as part of a normal and healthy metabolic process. This occurs just by living our daily lives – and it is not a big deal. As we age, deal with more stress, and have more and more free radical damage throughout the body, the cells start to increase their rate of being damaged more than ever.

This is where the process of autophagy comes into play. This is the natural process in the body that helps clear up damaged cells inside and includes cells that have gotten old and do not serve any functional purposes but haven't been removed out of organs and tissues yet. While it is natural for the body to get old and have damaged cells, it is not a good idea to have them stay around. You need to remove these cells because they can trigger inflammatory pathways and will end up contributing to a wide range of diseases as well.

The word 'autophagy' was coined more than forty years ago. It comes from the Greek words *auto*, which means self, and *phagy*, which means eating. Hence, basically, the body is going to be the process of self-eating. This may not sound like the best thing in the world; however, it is a natural and completely good thing to occur in your body. What this means is that the body is going to clean itself out, removing all the old and damaged cells, to allow more room for the healthy cells that you want to have there.

It has only been in the past few years that researchers have actually had a chance to observe the process of autophagy. What they have found is that autophagy can help promote longevity and provides a ton of benefits when it comes to your metabolism, heart, immune system, and nervous system. Let's take a more in-depth look at the process of autophagy and why it is such a great thing to implement into your own daily routine.

What Is Autophagy?

The first thing that we need to take a look at is the process of autophagy. The definition of autophagy is the consumption of the body's own tissues as a metabolic process occurring in starvation and in certain diseases – this is just a convoluted sentence which means that the body will use its own processes to eat up and remove tissues in the body. This process usually happens during fasting and when certain diseases occur. Researchers think that this is a type of survival mechanism or a way that the body can respond to stress in your life to keep itself protected.

The next thing to look at is whether autophagy is a bad thing or a good thing for your health. Autophagy is a *very* good thing for your life. As touched on earlier, autophagy is "self-eating of the body," which may sound a bit strange, but it is a completely healthy and normal way for the body to go through the cellular renewal process. In fact, autophagy is going to be so beneficial that it is seen as one of the biggest keys to preventing many common diseases, such as diabetes, cancer, liver disease, infections, and autoimmune diseases.

One of the first benefits that you will notice with autophagy is that it can help prevent many of the causes linked to aging. The reason that it is so successful with this is that it helps destroy and then reuse any damaged components that are likely to occur in the spaces within the cells. What this means is that autophagy is going to work by using the waste that the cells produce in order to create brand-new materials that are used for building up and repairing different parts of the body.

There are not many long-term studies about autophagy, but from some of the ones that have recently come out, we know that autophagy is important to clean up the body and defend against some of the negative effects that bother us due to stress in our modern world. However, the way that this works is something that is not completely understood yet, which could make it hard to understand why this is a process that is so necessary and beneficial. However, as more research is done, we will be able to learn more about the whole process and put it to more use for our needs.

A few different steps are involved when it comes to the autophagic process. First, lysosomes are the part of the cells that will go in and destroy large damaged structures, such as the mitochondria of the cells, and then take those damaged parts out of the cell, using them as a form of fuel. When the damaged cells are used as fuel, they can then be eliminated out of the body just like any other type of waste.

Without this autophagic process occurring, some issues can arise. The damaged and old cells and parts are just going to stick around the body, and they will never be able to clean themselves up. This makes it hard for the cells, and the parts they make up, to heal themselves. This can lead to inflammation, chronic diseases, and more.

How Was Autophagy Discovered?

Keith R. Porter and his student Thomas Ashford from the Rockefeller Institute were some of the first to observe the autophagic process. In January of 1962, they reported that they saw a higher number of lysosomes in rat liver cells after they added in glucagon to the diet and that some of these displaced lysosomes found near the center of the rat cells were holding onto other cell organelles like the mitochondria.

They called this process autolysis. However, Porter and Ashford were wrong about their interpretation of the data. They assumed that this was a part of lysosome formation. However, lysosomes can't be organelles in the cells since they are part of the cytoplasm, and the hydrolytic enzymes are going to be produced by the microbodies.

It was then in 1963 that Hruban, Spargo, and their colleagues were able to publish a very detailed description of what they were able to call 'focal cytoplasmic degradation'. This study was able to reference a study that was done in Germany in 1955 that looked at injury induced sequestration. This study recognized that there were three stages of maturation of the sequestered cytoplasm to lysosomes and that this process was not something that had to be limited to the body being injured. This was then the first time that the lysosomes of the cells were established as the main site and source of the autophagic process.

It wasn't until the 1990s, though, that a new era of research into autophagy began to take hold. During this time, there was more than one group of researchers whom all discovered genes that were related to autophagy using budding yeast, and all of these groups were able to do so independently. And then, in 2003, a unified nomenclature was advocated to list out the autophagy genes that had been discovered.

In 1999, there was a landmark discovery that linked autophagy and cancer. And, to date, this is still a major theme when it comes to researching autophagy. The roles of autophagy in immune defense and other neurological disorders have seen much attention over the years as well.

The idea of autophagy has definitely seen many changes throughout the years. While there is still much research that needs to be done concerning this topic and how it can benefit humans, there has already been a lot of interest in this topic throughout the world. Research that began over forty years ago is now being used to see how well autophagy can help with a bunch of different diseases and conditions of the body, and being able to work with this process and figure out how to induce this process, can ensure you prevent and keep away many different diseases of the body.

The Benefits of Autophagy

This chapter has discussed a bit about autophagy, but there are so many other benefits that come with the process. It is time to talk about them now. Some of the research that has been done concerning autophagy suggests that some of the benefits that you will find when you encourage this process include:

- Provides the cells with the energy and the building blocks that they need on a molecular level.
- Recycles all the damaged parts of the cells, including the organelles, proteins, and aggregates.
- Helps the mitochondria to regulate their own functions. When this happens, the cell can produce more energy and won't have to deal with as much damage from oxidative stress.
- Clears out the peroxisomes and the endoplasmic reticulum when they are damaged.
- Protects the nervous system better than anything else. It can also help by encouraging the nerve cells of the brain to grow more. Because of this, and other factors, it seems that autophagy can improve cognitive function, neuroplasticity, and brain structure.
- It helps support the growth of the cells in the heart and can protect against many diseases of the heart.
- Enhances the immune system to keep us feeling strong and healthy. It does this by getting rid of many pathogens that show up in the body.

- Defends against the misfolded and toxic proteins that will contribute to a variety of different diseases through the body.
- Can ensure that the stability of your DNA is protected. When DNA is damaged, it can make the genes behave in a way that is not natural. This can make you more predisposed to a variety of conditions that can be hard to deal with.
- Can prevent any unnecessary damage to the healthy organs and tissues of the body so they can continue with their own process.
- Can potentially help with a wide variety of other issues, including fighting cancer and dealing with neurodegenerative diseases. There still needs to be more research done to determine how and if autophagy can help fight cancer, but so far, the research looks promising, and this may be exactly what we need to help deal with the horrible disease.

There are also a few different types of autophagy that you may come across in your studies. Macroautophagy is the one that is talked about in this guidebook and is the most common. This type of autophagy is going to be known as an "evolutionarily conserved catabolic process involving the formation of vesicles that engulf the cellular macromolecules and organelles." To make it simple, this kind is basically the one that will find the damaged and old cells in the body, and then clean them all out so that the body will perform the way that you want it to.

What is interesting here is that humans are not the only species who can benefit from the process of autophagy. There are many other organisms too that will see this process happen, including mammals, flies, plants, mold, worms, and yeast. Most of the research that is out there about autophagy has been done with rats and yeast, but more and more studies are now being done to see how autophagy will affect humans and all of the great benefits that can come with this process in your life.

Is There a Relationship Between Autophagy and Apoptosis?

First, we need to understand what apoptosis is. Apoptosis is the death of cells that occurs as a normal and controlled part of the organism's growth or development. Researchers looking at autophagy believe that this process is going to be selective about what it is going to remove out of the body. There is not any clear evidence that either autophagy or apoptosis controls the other process, but some beginning studies do indicate that autophagy is a mechanism of apoptosis independent cell death.

One main reason that there is such an interest in this kind of relationship is that many researchers now believe that autophagy may be a process that, when used properly, could help treat many neurodegenerative diseases, and cancer, thanks to the ability of the process to modulate cell death. It is possible that autophagy can act kind of like a therapeutic target, ensuring that the harmful materials are removed, and protecting any cells that are considered healthy.

While there needs to be more research done to see how true this is and what can be done to make it more effective, it is possible that, in the future, we could use autophagy to protect all of the healthy cells that we do not want to die, and destroy and remove all of the cells that are damaged or diseased.

How Can I Induce Autophagy?

The third question that we need to ask at this point is how you can induce this process of autophagy. We already know that there are a ton of benefits of choosing this kind of process, and now you are probably wondering what you need to do to induce this process and see amazing results.

Autophagy is active in all cells, but it is going to be increased in response to stress or some kind of nutrient deprivation, such as starvation or fasting. This means that you can choose to work with good stressors in the form of exercise or with a temporary calorie restriction, such as fasting, to boost the autophagic processes. Both of these strategies have been linked to many good benefits, such as longevity, weight control, and the inhibition of many diseases that are associated with aging.

Let's take a look at some of the different methods that we can use to induce autophagy in your own life.

Practice fasting

When it comes to some of the lifestyle and diet habits that you can control, the thing that you can do that will trigger autophagy is fasting. You can even use the common dietary strategy that is called intermittent fasting. Fasting is a very simple concept. You will increase your fasting window while decreasing your eating window. You would still have a lot of liquids and waters, as long as they don't have any calories in them, to keep your body hydrated and help you get through the fast.

If you don't know about intermittent fasting, we will take a look at it a bit later on in more detail. However, intermittent fasting is cyclical fasting that will involve time-restricted eating. There are many different types of intermittent fasting, and all of them will be pretty effective – you just need to decide the method that works the best for you.

Now, you may be wondering how long you need to go on a fast for in order to achieve autophagy? Studies suggest that you should go on a fast that is between one to two days long to get the most benefits. However, this is a long time, and it isn't always the easiest for people to do. It is best to aim for at least a sixteen-hour fast in the beginning and see if you can build up from there. Even these shorter fasts can promote autophagy throughout the body.

An easy way to do one of these smaller fasts is to stick with just one or two meals a day, rather than three meals and a bunch of snacks. If you do end up finishing your dinner at about seven o'clock at night, then try not eating anything until eleven o'clock or noon the next day, and skipping breakfast in the process. This allows you to be on a fast that promotes autophagy, without feeling deprived in the process.

You can also choose to go on an occasional fast that lasts two to three days once you have time to gain more experience with fasting. If you do find that alternate day fasting works for you, then you need to restrict your calorie amount during the fasting days to either nothing, or do a variation that allows for 500 calories. Then, on the days that you are not fasting, make sure that you eat a healthy and nutritious diet to help support autophagy even more.

Fasting of all kinds can help you see results when you are trying to induce autophagy. You can choose to go on an extended water fast, which will take about seven to ten days, of only drinking water and avoiding food. Sometimes this may seem like a stretch for going on the fast, and most people will choose to only go on an intermittent fast – one that usually lasts for less than 36 hours overall. However, you can choose the type of fasting that most interests you, and then implement that into your own schedule in order to see the autophagic process show up in your life.

Think about going on the ketogenic diet

Another method that you can try to use to help promote the process of autophagy in your life is to consider going on the ketogenic diet. The ketogenic diet is a diet that is very low carb and very high fat and provides some of the same results in the body as fasting – without any fasting or longer periods of not eating. The keto diet is going to involve getting around 75 percent of your calories from fat each day, and no more than five percent of your calories out of carbs. The rest can come from moderate amounts of protein.

The reason that you would want to go with this kind of diet plan is because it changes up the metabolism in the body, forcing you to stop using the readily available glucose (which is almost gone now that you are limiting your intake so much), and has the body rely on healthy fats for fuel instead. This can help you to speed up the metabolism, burn the extra fat and weight hanging around the body, and make you feel better.

What are some of the most beneficial foods to use when you want to follow the ketogenic diet? You will want to go with foods that are whole and high in fat, such as nuts and seeds, avocado, fermented cheeses, grass-fed meat, ghee, butter, eggs, olive oil, and higher-fat choices of meat. Vegetables can be included, especially the ones that have a lot of fiber in them – as long as you keep the carb content in them as low as possible.

In response to limiting your carbs so much, you will see ketone bodies formed, and these are going to have many effects that protect various organs and tissues. Some studies suggest that this process of ketosis is also going to cause starvation-induced autophagy, which can help the body out in so many different ways.

For example, in one animal study that was done, rats were put on the ketogenic diet. In this study, the keto diet was able to start the autophagic pathways that reduced brain injury, both during and after seizures. This is definitely an area that is going to need more time and research in the future, but it can show just how great the ketogenic diet can be when you want to get the process of autophagy started in your body.

Exercise

Another one of the good stressors that you need to worry about when you want to start the autophagic process is exercise. Recent research shows how exercise can help to induce this process in several organs, especially the ones that are the most involved in regulating the metabolism, such as the adipose tissue, pancreas, liver, and muscles.

While many benefits come with exercise, it can be considered a form of stress because it will break down tissue throughout the body. These tissues need to be repaired so that they can grow back stronger than ever. Right now, studies are uncertain about how much exercise you will need to do in order to start or boost up autophagy. However, it is suggested that doing intense exercise can be the most beneficial to help you see these kinds of results.

When you are working on the muscle tissue that is cardiac and skeletal, you could find that just 30 minutes of exercise could be enough to induce autophagy. In addition, you could exercise while you are in one of the fasts as well, which helps you get even better results in the process.

Some Precautions to Consider About Autophagy and Fasting

There is still a lot that researchers need to find out concerning autophagy and how best to induce it or even boost it. Beginning to induce autophagy by incorporating fasting and regular exercise into your routine is often a fantastic place to start. Both of these things, especially when they are combined together, can provide the body with many benefits in addition to autophagy.

However, if you are on certain medications that are meant to help control different health conditions, it may be a good idea to talk to your doctor before you decide to get started on a fasting regiment. People who suffer from diabetes or hypoglycemia, and women who are either pregnant or breastfeeding, should never fast. Anyone who is dealing with or being treated for a disease, such as cancer, should make sure that they discuss this option with their doctor before starting as well.

There are so many great benefits to enjoy when it comes to the process of autophagy. This is a simple process that can really make a difference in your overall health and can stop many common diseases that seem to take over as we age and make us sick. Finding ways to induce or boost this process, such as through fasting, trying out diets like the ketogenic diet, or exercising, can ensure that the body cleans itself out and feels the very best.

Chapter 2: How Does It Work – The Science Behind What Happens to Our Bodies When We Fast

As mentioned in the previous chapter, fasting can be one of the main ways that you can enter the autophagic process, and it can be a great way to boost this process as well. Fasting allows the body to enter into a starvation mode for a bit, which can signal to the body that it is time to clean itself out of all the damaged and old parts and use them as fuel instead of relying on the food that we are used to enjoying.

The next question here is – what actually happens to our bodies when we go on a fast. Why is the process of autophagy so prevalent and work so efficiently to clear out the body, by only skipping a few meals along the way? Let's take a look at some of the things that will happen to your body when you decide to add fasting to your life and why it is so effective at helping you to start the process of autophagy.

About four or five hours after you are done eating, you will notice that the levels of insulin in your body are going to start falling. When these levels fall, this will trigger a series of hormonal changes because we start to enter into the fasting state. The first step here is that the body will use any readily accessible stores of glucose, or glycogen, to keep the body going and provide us with energy. After about ten to twelve hours, these stores are going to be depleted, and the body will begin to look for another source of fuel to keep it going. From there, the body will start to rely on stored fat in the body to keep itself going and full of energy.

The switch from glucose to fat as the biggest source of fuel in the body is key for many health benefits that come with fasting. It is going to take about twelve hours after your last meal before the body can use up all of the glucose stores that it has, and before it will start to use fat for energy. This is why you want to consider going on a 24-hour or longer fast. This ensures that you get at least twelve hours of fat burning out of the process. Of course, the amount of energy that you are going to derive from the excess stored body fat can vary between each person, and some of the things that it will depend on include:

- Whether you are metabolically flexible or fat adapted – what this means is whether your body is adapted to switching over to fat burning or not.

- How much glycogen is stored in the body – this will often depend on how many carbs you have eaten in your meals, and how much glycogen the muscles and liver can hold onto as well.

- How quickly you can deplete those glycogen sores – this is often going to depend on how active you can be during these fasting periods.

- Once the insulin levels throughout the body have had enough time to fall efficiently so that fat will start to release out of its stores, then your body can burn fat instead of glucose, and you can start to reap some of the benefits in the process.

How Will My Body Change When I Am on a Fast?

Now that we have taken some time to look at what fasting can do, and how important it is for the body to start relying on the stored body fat to get more energy, it is time to take a look at some of the ways that our bodies are going to change when we fast on a regular basis. You will be amazed at some of the dramatic changes that can happen in the body as the fasting time progresses. Some of the most dramatic changes include:

- The levels of blood glucose are going to fall, which means that the levels of insulin will decrease as well. The cells are going to detect that there is a decrease in these levels. This forces them to stop being in a growth phase, and they will enter into the repair phase.

- Blood glucose levels are going to be stopped from falling too low too quickly thanks to the liver. When these blood glucose levels start to go down, the liver is going to work to increase its own glucose production.

- As the levels of insulin continue to decrease, the cells are going to develop a bigger sensitivity to the effects of insulin. This means that over time, and with the right fasting method, it is possible that the individual could see a decrease in their insulin resistance and an improvement in their glucose tolerance test results.

- In addition, the decreases in both the blood glucose and insulin levels are going to be even bigger in those individuals who are dealing with diabetes when they get started.

- You will also see that the secretion of glucagon during this time is further going to encourage the fat burning that you want with fasting.

- The biggest changes in insulin and with fat burning are often going to occur sometime between eighteen and 24 hours of fasting. This is why the longer fast can sometimes be a better option since the benefits are going to multiply themselves.

- As the fasting time progresses, the liver will then start to produce ketones from stored body fat to provide us with fuel. As the ketone level starts to rise in the blood, the brain can take up these ketones for its own energy.

- Leptin levels are going to start to fall, reaching their greatest decline after 36 hours. This may mean that you feel more hungry during the first day to a day and a half on the fast, but then it may go down a bit.

- Another thing to notice is that the hormone activity of the thyroid is going to increase at first. Then after 24 to 36 hours, it is going to decrease. This is going to be accompanied by an initial increase in the rate of the metabolism, and then there will be a nice gradual decrease.

- Those who go on a fast will also notice that their total cholesterol and the HDL or high-density lipoprotein will rise during the fast. This is because fat is now being transported around the body as fuel and is not a big deal.

- The growth hormone production is going to head up during this time, which is a good way to encourage fat burning while also protecting the muscles, so they aren't broken down for glucose.

- You will see that the insulin-like growth factor levels will start to see a decrease as well.

- There will be some changes in the brain which are going to produce chemicals that enhance nerve growth and can bring about a sense of well-being.

These are all changes that you can see in your body when you decide to go on a fast. The longer fasts are more likely to see more of these benefits than others because the body has more time to show off these benefits. However, some changes are not going to happen as quickly or necessarily to the extent in those who are metabolically inflexible or those who are obese compared to those who have more tolerance and are more used to fasting, or those who are lean. It could take a few fasts in some individuals before these changes are instigated into your life smoothly.

As the body has some time to adapt to the fast, there are going to be a ton of benefits that come with it. We will talk about these in a bit, but you will see that a good fast can: reduce fat in the body, reduce the issues that can come with insulin resistance, which in turn decreases the risk of heart disease and diabetes, as well as a reduction in inflammation and disorders that come with these, and even the inhibition of cell growth, especially in cells that could be cancerous.

The Health Benefits of Fasting

When it comes to going on a fast, many different benefits can come with being on one. Many people don't realize the benefits that come with just a short fast, much less the number of benefits you will get if you decide to go on a longer fast. Let's take a look at some of the health benefits of fasting, and why it can be one of the best ways to see the changes that occur in your body thanks to fasting.

Can change the way that the hormones and cells function

When you spend more time not eating, there are a few different things that can happen to your body. To start, the body can initiate important cellular repair processes (namely the process of autophagy), and it can change up the hormone levels to ensure that stored body fat is easier to get to. There are a number of changes that will show up in your body while you are fasting that relate to this topic, and they include:

- Gene expression: There are going to be some changes in your molecules and genes when you go on a fast, especially the ones that are responsible for protecting you against diseases and helping you to live longer.
- Cellular repair: The body is going to induce many different repair processes on a cellular level when you are on a fast. This can include removing any material that is considered waste from the cells.
- Human growth levels: The levels of growth hormone found in the blood could increase by five times when you are fasting. These higher levels of the growth hormone help with a gain in muscle and fat burning, as well as providing you with many other benefits.
- Insulin levels: You will find that on a fast, the levels of insulin in the blood can drop quite a bit, which will facilitate fat burning.

You will see weight loss

One of the benefits of autophagy, as well as fasting, is weight loss. Unless you spend a lot of time overcompensating for the amount of time that you weren't eating, it is possible that you will lose some weight. There are a number of reasons for this. For example, having lower levels of insulin and higher levels of growth hormone can help you break down fat in the body easier, and you can use this as energy. Because of this, short-term fasting can increase your metabolism by up to fourteen percent, making it easier to burn even more calories than before.

Fasting can work on both sides of this calorie equation. You will find that it will boost your metabolic rate, which means that it increases the number of calories that go out. Fasting can also do wonders by reducing how much food you eat during your eating times, unless you go crazy, which can reduce the calories that you take in.

Can reduce inflammation and oxidative stress throughout the body

As many studies are showing, oxidative stress is actually one of the main steps towards chronic diseases and aging. What happens with this is that unstable molecules, which go by the name of free radicals, get into the body. These free radicals are not supposed to be there, and they are very good at reacting with some of the other important molecules, like your DNA and protein, and causing much damage to them.

There are numerous studies out there that show how intermittent fasting can actually help the body become more resistant to this oxidative stress. In addition to this, fasting can help fight off inflammation, which is another problem for many common diseases that are associated with aging and a poor diet.

Can help keep your heart health

Heart disease is considered one of the biggest killers throughout the world. And because there are so many risk factors out there that can cause heart disease, it is no wonder that we need to always be on the lookout to ensure our hearts stay as strong and healthy as possible.

It is commonly known that there are different risk factors or health markers that are associated with either an increase or a decrease in your risk of developing heart disease. Fasting is known to help improve several of the risk factors. Some of the ways that fasting can help is by lowering blood pressure and helping with blood sugar levels, blood triglycerides, LDL cholesterol, and inflammatory markers.

This one will need to have a bit more research done on it before we can know for sure. A lot of the information about how effective fasting can be on our heart health is based on animal studies. However, it stands to reason that if you stick with the protocols that come with your fasting method, you will increase the metabolism and burn off more of that excess body fat, which is seen as one of the biggest risk factors to heart disease. Add in a healthy diet when you do eat, and you will see a big difference in your health.

Can help with a variety of repair processes in the cells

When we fast, the cells that are inside the body are going to start the autophagic process in order to get rid of all the wastes in the cells. This is going to involve the cells getting broken down and then being metabolized. This ensures that all of these old and damaged parts of the cells are broken down and then sent out of the body to keep you healthier. Increasing the autophagy that occurs in the body may protect against many different types of disease, such as cancer and Alzheimer's.

You can see changes in your brain health

Anything that provides many benefits to the body will also provide many benefits to the brain. Fasting has been known to improve a lot of other features of the metabolism that are also important for the health of your brain. This could include a reduction in oxidative stress, a reduction in the amount of inflammation in the body, and even a reduction in the resistance to insulin and blood sugar levels.

There have been different studies done that show how intermittent fasting may increase the growth of new nerve cells, which is going to have a ton of benefits for how well the brain can function. It is also going to increase the number of BDNF (brain-derived neurotrophic factor). When there is a deficiency of this, it could be a cause of depression and other problems of the brain.

Can help extend your lifespan and help you live longer than before

One of the best parts of being on a fast is that it can help extend your lifespan if you follow it properly. There have been several studies done that show how fasting in all forms can extend your lifespan in a similar way to what has been seen with continuous calorie restriction. In addition, some of these studies showed that the effects of the fast were very dramatic. In fact, one of these studies showed that the rats who went on a fast every alternate day were able to live up to 83 percent longer compared to the rats who didn't fast at all.

While more studies still need to be done on this (it is hard to measure longevity in humans because of how long they live to start with), fasting is definitely something that has become popular among those who favor anti-aging. And given the fact that there are many metabolic benefits of fasting, and all of the benefits of other health markers with fasting, it does make sense that this could be the right tool to help you live a healthier, and longer, life.

There are so many benefits that come with going on a fast. It can help the body to remove much of the waste that it has inside. It can help us to feel younger and can prevent aging. And it even helps with weight loss, the functioning of the brain, and so much more. When it comes to implementing the process of autophagy, something that is very much a part of all these things, fasting is one of the best methods to use to see a ton of results.

Special Considerations for Women Who Want to Use Fasting

Now that we have introduced the idea of fasting, it is time to look specifically on how fasting can work for women. It is important that women understand that they need to handle the fast a bit differently than men. Some women can go on any of the fasting protocols we list here, and they won't have any problems at all. However, others may find that fasting is too extreme, or they need to take it slowly to see how their bodies react, rather than jumping right in.

Many women do experience some issues when it comes to fasting. They can see their metabolism slow down, issues with their reproductive system, fewer or no periods, and even early menopause. This is why it is so important for women to take some extra precautions when they want to go on any type of fast for their health.

To keep this simple, it seems that going on a fast, especially some of the longer-term fasts, can cause a hormonal imbalance for some women, especially if they are not careful and they don't go on the fast properly. Women and their hormones seem to be extremely sensitive, at least more so than men, to any signals of starvation in the environment. If the body feels as if it is being starved, it is going to start ramping up its own production of ghrelin and leptin, which are the hunger hormones in the body.

So, when women go on a fast and start to feel overly hungry after they under-eat, they are experiencing this process happening. Their hormones are increasing, and this causes them to be hungry – this is basically the female body trying to protect a potential fetus, even if you are not pregnant or have no plans to become pregnant in the near future.

When you continue on the fast and try to ignore these intense hunger cues, it just makes them worse. Often we fail and binge later on, before following all of that up with some more undereating and starvation again in the hopes that we can finally get it right. It is this vicious cycle that throws the hormones out of control, and if care is not taken, it may cause the halt to ovulation in some women.

In some animal studies that have been done, after two weeks of an intermittent fast, the female rats stopped having their menstrual cycles, and there was shrinkage in the ovaries. In addition, these female rats experienced more insomnia compared to their male counterparts. The men did suffer a little with lower testosterone production while fasting but did not see as dramatic effects as women.

Right now, there are not as many human studies that have been done to look at the differences between how women and men do on these kinds of fasts, but if the animal studies we look at can confirm anything, it is that going on this kind of fasting for too long could throw off the hormonal balance in some women. This could cause issues like fertility problems and may make various eating disorders like binge eating, bulimia, and anorexia more prevalent as well.

If you don't go on a fast properly, it can be hard on the body, especially if you are new to the whole idea, or you jump into it without proper preparation. So, if you are a woman and it is your first time doing any fast, you may find that doing a modified version of fasting, or a crescendo fasting, will work the best for you. This helps the body ease into the fasting regimen, which can make it easier for the body to adjust without feeling like it is going into starvation.

With crescendo fasting, you only need to do a fast a few days each week, rather than trying to do it every day. This is a great way for you to get the benefits of fasting without accidentally throwing your hormones out of place. If you find that you can do this kind of fasting without any issues, then you can increase the amount of time, or the number of days, that you go on a fast. This method is easier and gentler and helps the body adapt better to the fasting regimen without problems.

Not all women are going to need to start with a crescendo fasting, but it can definitely be a good option to go with. It ensures that you are going to see success, and gently eases the body into the fasting regimen without having anything be overdone in the process.

Now, the rules that come with crescendo fasting are pretty easy to follow, and you will find that the fasting periods aren't as long and you still feel some of the benefits that come with it. Some of the rules that you should follow when it comes to crescendo fasting include:

> 1. Pick out two or three nonconsecutive days during the week that you will go on a fast. You may choose to do Tuesday, Thursday, and Saturday if you want to work with three days, for example.

2. On the fasting days, you can do a bit of exercise, but make sure it is something simple and not too strenuous. Try out a nice walk around the block or some yoga.

3. For these fasts, you do not want to go for a long period of time. Twelve to sixteen hours is usually enough to get the results you want and ease your body into the process of fasting.

4. On the other days of the week, eat normal and healthy diets. You can also do HIIT (high-intensity interval training) or strength training on these days to help keep you active.

5. Make sure that you drink plenty of water, especially during the fasting period. It is fine to have some coffee or tea on occasion to mix things up, just don't add in any sweetener or milk.

6. After two to three weeks, evaluate how you are feeling. If you feel that things are going well and you can handle more, go ahead and add in another day of fasting to your week.

7. An optional thing that you can try out when you go on this crescendo fasting is to take about five to eight grams of BCAAs during the fast. These are known as branched chain amino acids and taking this supplement does have a few calories, but not enough to throw you off your fast. This is going to provide some extra fuel to your muscles so you can stay strong while fasting, and it helps to take the edge off fatigue and hunger.

Going on the crescendo fast is not something that everyone has to do. And if you feel that another form of fasting is better for you, then go ahead and try it out. There is no one-size-fits-all when it comes to the world of fasting and seeing results from autophagy, which is why there are so many protocols that you can choose from.

However, because some women are very sensitive to changes in food and the environment, it is not always best to jump right into fasting. This can mess with the system and make it hard to keep things in line. Working with an easier fast, such as the crescendo fast, can ensure that you get the benefits of this fast, without having to worry about the negative side effects that could come from your hormones getting messed up.

Everyone can benefit from a little fasting in their lives. Whether you decide to go all out and try to work alternate day fasting or you want to ease into it with one of the other methods we will talk about you will find that there are a ton of benefits that come with this eating strategy.

Chapter 3: Myths vs. Truths – Common Misconceptions About Autophagy and Fasting

Before we get into more information about fasting and what it all entails, it is important to dispel some of the common myths and misconceptions that can come with the idea of fasting and autophagy. These misconceptions are going to make it hard to convince some people that going on a fast is actually a good idea. We have spent years hearing about how we need to eat every few hours and that skipping meals is such a bad thing for us – when, in reality, it can help to speed up our metabolisms and the process of autophagy.

Let's take a look at some of the most common myths that are out there about fasting and autophagy and come to understand why they are instead really good for our overall health.

Fasting Is Going to Put Your Body in Starvation Mode

One common misconception that many people will have when it comes to going on a fast is that fasting will put you into starvation mode. Starvation mode is the period in your body where the metabolism shuts down to conserve energy because you have gone a long time without food. If starvation mode occurs too much, it can mess with the metabolism and make weight loss almost impossible.

However, for the most part, unless you do something really off with your fast, you will see some amazing benefits when you go on a fast, without ever having to worry about going into starvation mode at the same time. Most research shows that it takes at least 72 hours before starvation mode becomes a big problem for most people. Since many people decide that they will stick with intermittent fasting, they will be on and off the fast before these issues even come up.

Even if you do go on a longer fast, as long as you aren't fasting all of the time, and you eat a healthy diet beforehand, you don't have to worry about starvation mode. Starvation mode is only going to be an issue when the individual decides to go on a fast for a very long time, or they go too extreme with their fasting rules. For example, if you go on a two-week fast every month and then cut your calories down to 800 for the rest of the month, you are probably not giving the body the nutrients it needs. If you go on a twenty-hour fast each day, and then only eat 500 calories after that, then there are issues as well.

The most important thing to remember about starvation mode is that the body needs to feel that it is really short on nutrients and that it is likely not to get those nutrients soon. It goes into this mode as a way to deal with the lack of nutrients. If you keep your fasts reasonable, and make sure that you take in enough calories each day, or overall, with healthy and nutritious foods, then you can enjoy going on a fast and experiencing the autophagic process, without having to worry about starvation mode.

Fasting Is Going to Make You Overeat and Can Ruin the Effects of Autophagy

One common concern that comes up when we talk about fasting and autophagy is the idea that once you are done with the fast, you are going to overeat, and then all of the benefits will be canceled out. It is true that you are going to be incredibly hungry when you are done with fasting; however, this doesn't mean that you have to give in to those cravings and those urges along the way.

This is where some planning needs to come in. You may have the best resolution in the world to not overeat and to stay healthy and get all of the benefits from fasting, but then you go some time without eating, and you get hungry. When your eating window finally opens again, you are going to be really hungry, and your body will crave everything sweet and unhealthy. Without some planning, it is possible that you will end up overeating.

This doesn't mean that you are counteracting all the benefits of the autophagy that occurred during that time. However, it is something that you need to work on a bit. Meal planning can definitely be the answer that you are looking for if you decide to go on a fast to help with weight loss as well.

When you come up with a meal plan, consider adding a few extra calories into the beginning meal, or the first one that you have after you finish the fast. And perhaps consider having a healthier "treat" on there. In the beginning, you are going to have cravings, and they will be hard to deal with. And you are going to be hungry. Don't ignore this. Rather than trying to split up the calories completely evenly when you have three meals after the fast, give the first meal some extra calories, and cut the others down a little bit. This helps you to eat a little extra and satisfy those cravings, while also ensuring that you aren't going to feel deprived.

Fasting Is Bad for Your Health

If you read the previous chapter, you know that it is not true that fasting is bad for your health. We have had some long-held beliefs that fasting is a horrible thing for our bodies. We assume that it is going to put our bodies into starvation mode, that we are going to feel miserable, and that we will have such a slow metabolism from missing even one meal that we can kiss losing weight goodbye forever.

But does any of this really make sense? Does it make sense that we would enter starvation mode just from missing a meal or two? Our ancestors didn't have a ton of food just sitting around, and they may have had to go several days without getting any good at all. Does this mean that they went into starvation mode and their metabolisms were ruined all the time?

Have you ever been sick and had to go a few days without eating? Whether you were just suffering from the flu and didn't have anything to eat for a few days, or you were throwing up and couldn't keep anything down, we have all gone without eating during that time as well. Did that mean we entered into starvation mode and our metabolisms were ruined forever?

Of course not. Our bodies are designed to take a little bit of stress, and missing a meal here or there is not a big deal. Studies and research have shown that you can go up to 72 hours on a fast before the big side effects of starvation mode start to become an issue. And as long as you make sure that your diet is full of healthy and nutritious foods when you are no longer fasting, it is easy to add in the daily, or a few times a week, fasts that are common with intermittent fasting.

If you can add one of the protocols of fasting into your routine, you are going to get a whole host of benefits out of the process. You will get to enjoy a healthier heart, weight loss, mental clarity, better blood pressure, fewer issues with insulin resistance and diabetes, and so much more – all it takes it putting the body on a short fast on occasion and allowing the process of autophagy to take control.

Fasting and Autophagy Will Burn Off Muscles

Studies that take a look at alternate daily fasting show that the concern over losing muscle on a fast is misplaced. Alternate daily fasting over a period that was 70 days long did see a decrease in body weight of an average of six percent in participants. However, the fat mass of those same individuals did increase by eleven point four percent. But the lean mass, which includes muscle and bone, didn't see any changes at all.

In addition, there were big improvements that were seen in the LDL (low-density lipoprotein) and triglyceride levels. The growth hormone increased, which was important in helping the participants maintain their muscle mass. To take this even further, some studies show that eating just one meal each day resulted in a significant amount of fat loss, even if that meal included the same number of calories as eating three or more times during the day. The most important thing here, though, is that there was no evidence of muscle loss at all.

Let's take this even further. More recently, a randomized trial of fasting versus caloric restriction found that there really wasn't any evidence that muscle was burned up during the fasting process. During this same trial, the fasting group was told to follow the 36-hour fasting protocol every other day, also known as alternate day fasting. This shows great promise for those who want to get started on fasting for all of the health benefits, but who were scared about the loss in muscle that may result.

According to some experts who seem not to look at the studies above, fasting will burn off 1/3 of a pound of muscle each day that you are on it. What this results in is about 1 pound of muscle a week if you go on an alternate-day fast. This also means that you would see a reduction of 32 pounds of muscle in a group that does fasting for 32 weeks.

However, the actual amount that the fasting group lost over 32 weeks was about 2.6 pounds or 1.2 kg. Yes, this was a little bit of muscle weight loss, but when it was compared to the participants who just went on a calorie restriction, it was less. Those participants who simply restricted their calories ended up losing 16 kg during that same period.

It makes sense that a bit of lean mass is going to be lost when you lose weight. You are losing some of the extra skin and connective tissue at the same time, but the lean mass percentage actually does increase by about 22 percent when you are on a fast.

As you can see, fasting does not burn off a ton of muscle mass, and it won't make you a weak person who is going to suffer from metabolism issues for the rest of your life because you no longer have any muscle mass to deal with. And if you are worried about the slight amount of muscle mass that is lost (which is still less than what you would see with just going on a calorie restriction), then consider adding in some strength training or weight training to your routine to help.

You Can't Exercise When You Are on a Fast

Another misconception is the idea that you are not allowed to work out when fasting. While it is true that you may have to go through and make some adjustments to the way that your workout compared to your normal routine, this doesn't mean that you aren't allowed to work out at all.

When you go on a fast, you are working to deplete the stores of glycogen that are in the body so that you start relying more on the stored fat. During this process, the body may feel a little bit tired and worn down. It is so used to getting the glycogen on a regular basis, and that is a much easier source of fuel for it to rely on than the stored fat. The body will feel weak and worn down for a few days, and sometimes even later on as it adjusts to the fasting regimen.

Because of this, you may need to make some changes to the way that you exercise. Doing the workout right at the beginning of the fast can help because it ensures that you still have some glucose floating around the body to give you energy. Switching to something like HIIT training or weight lifting can be a nice way to ensure that you are still getting a good workout, that you are working on building and maintaining those strong muscles, and that you see even better results from both the fast and autophagy.

Autophagy Means We Have to Overstress Our Bodies

When it comes to autophagy, it is true that the body needs to undergo some stress to make the process happen. This is critical to assuring that the body will start to break down the old parts and build up new ones. If there is no breaking down, then how will there be room for the new cells and parts that you need?

This doesn't mean that we have to overstress our bodies and go crazy. Doing workouts that last six or seven hours each day and are incredibly intense, or fasting for a month straight may seem like they will help out more, but you will find that there are actually more effective, and easier, methods for starting the body on this process.

Simple exercise, such as an intense 30-minute workout or HIIT training, can be enough to help when you are looking to enter into autophagy. Going on a fast that is a few days long, or even just a one-day fast, can be enough to get the body started with autophagy. And these are much easier to start and maintain compared to the more intense options above. Autophagy needs a bit of stress to get started, but that doesn't mean that you have to go crazy in order to see the results.

Autophagy can be a great process for your whole body. It ensures that the body can function properly because it gets all of those old cells and proteins and other parts, and removes them so that new ones can start. It is a simple concept to work with, but you will find that it really does make a difference throughout your whole body.

Chapter 4: Two Ways to Water Fast

Now that we have spent a bit of time talking about the benefits of fasting, it is now time to look at the different methods of fasting that you have available at your disposal. There are two main types of fasting: intermittent and extended.

When we talk about intermittent fasting, we are usually talking about fasts that will last for about 24 hours or less – though sometimes they will go for a little bit longer. These are short fasts that you can implement into your daily routine and still provide you the benefits of autophagy that you are looking for, without having as big of a challenge.

When we are talking about extended fasting, it usually means a fast that lasts between seven to ten days. These fasts may pose more of a challenge since you are going without food and any calories for at least seven days. However, the benefits that you can get out of these fasts are amazing and can really ensure that autophagy has the time it needs to be successful.

Let's take a closer look at the way that these two fasting styles work so that you can decide which one is the best for you!

What Is Intermittent Fasting?

Intermittent fasting has become very popular as a way to help manage calories and lose weight, without all of the counting and other concerns that come with a traditional dieting plan. There are also many different protocols that come with it, which makes it easier for individuals to get on the fast and find the one that works the best for them.

When it comes to intermittent fasting, you are going to learn how to extend out the periods of not eating during the day, and limit how much time you are allowed to eat from one day to the next. It really is as simple as that. As long as you are careful about the foods that you are eating and you stick with your periods for eating, you will find that it is easier than ever to get weight loss and health benefits with intermittent fasting.

There are a variety of different methods that you can choose to go with when it comes to starting your own intermittent fast. The most common method is the 16/8 method. For this, you will limit your eating window to just eight hours a day, and then the rest of the day you rely on water and other non-caloric beverages to keep you hydrated. This is as simple as finishing your evening meal and not having any late-night snacks and then skipping breakfast the next day. Different variations come with this method, but they all basically change up how many hours you are allowed to eat and how many you should fast for. The goal is to make the fasting window bigger than the eating window.

Another method that is similar to the 16/8 fast is the warrior diet. For this, you will basically just have water and other non-caloric beverages for twenty hours of the week. You are allowed to have small amounts of fruits and vegetables during that fasting period, but try to keep these under 200 calories as a total. For the final four hours, you can eat one or two bigger meals to help you get the nutrition that the body needs to stay healthy.

The warrior diet can be hard to go on, especially since it is a fasting regimen that is supposed to happen every day of the week. Many people start out with some of the smaller fasting lengths and then build up to this, or just implement this period into their routine on occasion. You can mix and match to find the method that seems to work the best for you.

The 5:2 diet is another option that works well with intermittent fasting. When you go on this version, you will pick two days that you will fast on. These can be any two days of the week, as long as they are not right next to each other. So going on a fast on Tuesday and Thursday is fine under this kind of protocol. During those two days, you need to keep your calories at no more than 500 for women and 600 for men. You can choose how you would like to divide up the calories based on your own needs. Some people will split these calories into two different meals, and some like to wait until the end of the day and have all of the calories at the same time to help them not go to bed hungry. For the other five days of the week, you are required to eat a diet that is healthy and full of nutrition to help the body out.

Alternate day fasting is a popular method as well. For this one, you will go on a fast every other day. Some protocols ask you to go on a complete water fast, and others are fine if you choose to add in up to 500 calories. These can sometimes be turned into a 36-hour fast pretty easily as well. You should decide whether you are going to add in the calories or not, and then do some meal planning because this kind of fasting method can be intense.

The eat stop eat method is a nice one to choose as well. For this, you are going to get on a 24-hour fast. You will eat normally one day, stop eating for 24 hours, and then go back to eating normally. This one doesn't have to be as hard as it sounds. Simply stop eating after dinner one night, and then wait until dinner the next day before you eat again. This would give you a 24-hour fast and all of the benefits that come with it.

There is also the crescendo fasting that we talked about in a previous chapter. This is a good way for you to adjust your eating habits and get used to the new eating plan. You may find that intermittent fasting is quite a bit different than the eating plan that you are currently on. Many Americans are going to spend almost every waking moment eating. They start their day off with some breakfast, eat at lunch and dinner, and have a few snacks along the way. Going from eating all of this down to a more restricted eating window can be tough for anyone. The crescendo fasting, as well as other options, will help you deal with this by having you just fast a few times a week for shorter periods so that you can build up to some of the other fasting types.

There is not necessarily an eating plan that comes with intermittent fasting. You are allowed to eat whatever diet you would like when you are out of your fasting times. The thing here is that if you are not careful with the foods that you consume, then you will still end up gaining weight and not see the results that you want, even if you do go on this kind of fast.

As long as you eat meals that are healthy and full of nutrition, you are going to be amazed at the results that you can get with intermittent fasting. If you are looking for a method that seems to work really well, and many people are combining with their fasts, then you may want to go with the ketogenic diet as your eating plan.

The ketogenic diet is a low carb, high fat, moderate protein diet plan. It can help you to feel full and satisfied, which makes the fasting times easier to handle. In addition, it forces the body to enter into the process of ketosis faster than before, intensifying the results that you are trying to get when you go on a fast.

All of the methods of intermittent fasting can be very effective. Some of the methods that may be considered a bit easier are going to show results a little slower, but then you won't struggle on them as much. Some of the other methods that may pose more of a challenge, such as alternate day fasting, will provide you with the benefits even faster.

Make sure that you thoroughly research the fasting method that you want to go on before you get going. Each of the protocols will ask for slightly different rules, and it is important that you know the rules that go with your chosen fast. The good news is that these protocols, even though they go on a shorter fasting window than the extended fasts, can still show you many great health benefits over time, and they are easier to maintain over the long term.

Many people have decided that intermittent fasting is the right option for them. First, they can get many of the same benefits from going on an intermittent fast as they can with the extended fasts, plus these smaller fasts are often going to be much easier to handle. If you only have to do a few hours of fasting on a daily basis, or one or two all day fasts a week, it is much easier to handle than trying to go on a fast for a week or longer.

There are also many different options when it comes to starting an intermittent fast. You can choose which protocol you like the best, and you will get results from it. Some protocols are easier than others, which makes them perfect for any level of faster you are. If you are a beginner and a little nervous about getting started, then you can always start with a smaller daily fast and build up as you want. If you have done dieting for some time, or you need to heal some serious health conditions quickly, then you may want to consider going on one of the tougher fasts, such as the 5:2 or the alternate day fast.

Adding intermittent fasting into your day can be really easy. You may even pick out a certain protocol based on what works best for your schedule. And you don't have to worry about taking time off from work to rest because most of these fasts aren't going to wear you out as much as the extended fast will do. So, if you have one or two days at work that are really busy and you barely have time to eat on those days anyway, consider doing the 5:2 method and not eating until the end of the day for your 500 calories. If you barely have time to eat breakfast, consider going on the 16/8 fast plan and stop eating after supper and don't have breakfast in the morning.

It is super easy to start on an intermittent fast, and there are a ton of options out there to help you get in the best health and feel amazing. You just have to decide which method you want to go with and then get started!

What Is Extended Fasting?

Another form of fasting that you may want to try out is an extended fast. While intermittent fasting usually doesn't go much above 36 hours in most cases, although there are times when it may go up to 72 hours, an extended fast is going to work to make you fast for a longer period. Most of the extended water fasts will go somewhere between seven and ten days depending on the goals of the person following it and the amount of willpower and determination that they have. In some cases, the extended fast may last for fourteen days or a little longer, but these lengths are usually done under the supervision of a medical professional.

Fasting can provide the individual with clarity, increase how productive they are, and even extend their lifespan if used properly. Two main benefits come with fasting, and both of them can help your body heal itself and function much better than before. The first benefit is autophagy, which we have discussed in-depth in this guidebook and is the process that occurs naturally in the body where old cells are recycled, and new ones are created. The second main benefit of fasting is ketosis, which is when the body starts to use its own natural fat stores to help keep you energized.

Going somewhere between seven to ten days without any food and only enjoying water may seem a bit crazy, but this is the practice that is known as extended fasting, and it has become very popular. It is a method that will help you to challenge yourself a bit, but the rewards and the payoff are definitely worth all of the hard work. There are even a bunch of different gadgets and other pieces of technology that you can try out to track your different vital signs and make sure that you are doing well.

Extended fasting is going to be a bit different than intermittent fasting, but it can provide you with many of the same benefits that you are used to if you ever went on that kind of fast. Because of intermittent fasting, many different protocols have come up that are considered fasts. You can go on one that has you fast a few days a week, as long as you don't do those days consecutively. Some will have you not eat anything after supper and then not eat breakfast the next day. Research has shown that for at least some people, some great health benefits can come for most individuals who follow these kinds of eating patterns.

However, extended fasting is a bit different. Technically, extended fasting is going to be any fast that goes for more than 24 hours, but since some of the intermittent fasting protocols fall into this kind of category, it has been expanded to cover a fast that usually lasts a week to ten days. This kind of fasting works similarly and is going to provide you with some of the same benefits as your intermittent fasting – but it does belong to a different category because it is considered much more extreme compared to the other methods of fasting we have discussed.

Instead of missing out on a meal here or there, extended fasting takes away your solids for up to a week. Many people choose to go on an extended fast to help them lose weight, but this may not be the goal for everyone. Some people like the amount of mental clarity they can get when they go on an extended fast – and others want a quick fix to help them deal with some of their major health concerns.

If you are looking to lose weight, improve your concentration and focus, and help yourself reach an optimal level of health, then extended fasting may be the best choice for you. And a water fast during this time can help you feel hydrated and provide you with a ton of great benefits. Many people have gone on an extended water fast to improve their high blood pressure, solve issues with weight, help with insulin sensitivity, and so much more.

It is common to find that many of the individuals who do extended fasting are men, but there is a growing number of women jumping on board for this system as well. There are also different protocols that you can follow with this, and some people decide to build up to it, maybe starting with some of the different methods of intermittent fasting until they can build themselves up to the longer fasts of a week.

There is no denying that any kind of a fast, whether it is for one day, one week, or even longer, can bring about some side effects that are pretty unpleasant, especially for someone who is new to the idea. You are going to feel hungry during this time because your stomach is missing out on food. However, if you can keep yourself hydrated and find ways to distract yourself (as well as relaxing when needed), some of these issues will pass – other common side effects that may come up include headaches, trouble with sleeping, heartburn, irritability, and brain fogs. Even those who do this kind of fasting all the time now will state that this kind of extended fast can be hard until you gain some more familiarity with it.

It is going to be hard to get started with this long of a fast, but if you eat a diet that is healthy, both before and after the fast, you can still provide your body with the nutrients it needs to do well, and you can get all of the benefits of these longer fasts. Once you have done the fasts a few times, you will adjust and find many of the side effects dissipating and not bothering you as much. Just make sure that you take some breaks between your week-long fasts, so you give your body time to stock up on healthy nutrients and give it time to heal from the autophagy.

For your first extended fast, it may be best to stick with a time limit that is between five to seven days. You can always expand out later if you decide that this is the right choice for you. However, if you are not used to fasting, then it can be hard to take on more time than that for the first few opportunities that you get with it.

If you decide that going on an extended water fast is the right option for you, then it is time to get started. For this to work, you need to pick out the day and timeframe that you want to use for the fast. You get some freedom here, but it may be best, at least for the first few fasts, if you chose to just do it on days that you have off, or days that you can take off. You are going to feel a bit tired and worn out when you get started with the fast. While these will fade off after a few days, it is a good idea to give your body some time to rest and relax as it adjusts to the new fasting regimen.

You also need to make sure that you keep plenty of water nearby when you are on one of these longer fasts. Many people forget that even though they are not eating, they still need to take the time to drink plenty of water to keep themselves hydrated. Remember that not only do you need to drink the amount that was required before you went on the fast, but you are also missing out on about twenty percent of your daily water from the foods you usually eat, so add that in as well. Some of the worst side effects happen because you aren't getting hydrated enough, so work on preventing this problem from the beginning.

During this time, make sure that you find ways to distract yourself. Your hunger and lack of food situation will become a whole lot worse if you allow yourself to sit around and only focus on that. Consider finding some books to read, going out with some friends and doing something that is not food related – go on a walk, or binge watch some of your favorite shows. Just make sure that you are busy. You may even find, just like other people who go on an extended fast, that it actually feels pretty good to be up and moving and that you can get more done more productively.

Make sure that you listen to your body during this time. Some people can do the seven days and feel fine, although a bit hungry at the end. However, others may get to day four or day five and start to feel sick. They may not be drinking enough water or dealing with a serious complication. If you feel that something is wrong, make sure you go and visit your doctor right away.

While there are some risks for going on an extended fast, and these risks can be really important to watch out for if you are dealing with certain medical conditions, most people have decided that the payoffs are worth it all. The biggest thing to watch out for, during this kind of fast, is your own medical conditions. And if you are doing this just to lose weight quickly, then the weight is likely to come back. If you are using it as a way to improve your overall health and make you feel amazing, then this can be a great fast to go on.

You also need to be careful of the different health issues that can come up. While fasting can be very good for the body, having many periods where the body isn't getting calories can be hard on the body. For women, in particular, you have to be careful about how it could disrupt your hormones, cause insomnia, cause brain fog, and increase anxiety. Add to this that, in some cases, extended fasting can cause a reduction in fertility, and it is important to take precautions as a woman when going on one of these longer fasts.

For those who have certain medical conditions, or who are just a bit worried about how the fasting works and they want to be extra careful, doing this kind of fast under the supervision of a medical professional may be best. As long as you are not trying to conceive, and aren't nursing or pregnant, these fasts can go very well. In addition, those who are dealing with insulin-dependent diabetes, adrenal fatigue, and thyroid problems can benefit from having a medical professional watch over them as they go through the fasting.

When it comes to promoting the process of autophagy, you will find that both of these methods of fasting can be very effective and provide you with a ton of benefits in the process. Some find that they like going on the extended fasts because they provide the most benefits in a short amount of time, and can make one feel great. For others, they may find that going on a longer fast is just too hard for them to manage, and they can benefit from the shorter bursts of fasting that are prominent with intermittent fasting.

Chapter 5: Important to Note –
Things to Consider When You
Start Fasting

At this point, you may be ready to jump in and get started with your fasting. There are many benefits, and fasting is one of the best and fastest ways for you to enter into the process of autophagy. You know the benefits, you are excited to see what will happen, and you are ready to get the most out of fasting and all it has to offer.

However, there are a few aspects that you need to consider so that you can get the most out of this kind of eating plan.

Some of the Negative Side Effects

Many great benefits come with fasting, and we have talked about quite a few of them already in this guidebook. However, there are a few side effects that can occur when you first get started with fasting. These are pretty mild, and most of them are going to go away when you are used to fasting for a few weeks. Some of the negative side effects that you need to be aware of when you get started with any type of fasting include:

Hunger and cravings

These may not seem like a big deal, but when you are dealing with the fast and get to the end of it, your hunger and cravings will become crazy and be the only thing that you think about with fasting.

Of course, when you are done with a fast, you are going to feel hungry. You have gone for a long time without eating anything. Your stomach is going to be empty, and the body will want to eat something in order to feel better. The only way to deal with this hunger is to eat something. As soon as the fast is done, you can have a meal, and this side effect will go down. After some time, the body will be able to adjust to the fasting, and you won't feel as hungry. Until that time comes, find ways to distract yourself so that you don't focus on the hunger as much.

You may also notice that you have a lot of intense cravings when it comes to being on a fast. Your body wants to get that glucose back, and so if you are not careful when you are done with the fast, you may give in to these cravings and eat more than usual.

It is fine to give in to those cravings on occasion, especially right after the fast is done. This helps you to satisfy that craving rather than ignoring it and makes you feel less deprived. Just make sure that you work on a meal plan and include that craving into the first meal, rather than just letting your cravings go crazy. This helps you to stay within your calorie recommendations and makes it easier to see the results that you want without going overboard.

Heartburn and bloating

Your stomach is still going to produce a lot of acids, even when you stop eating for a bit, and this acid is so important for helping you digest food. On a traditional diet, you will often eat every few hours or more. This causes the body to get into the habit of producing acid every few hours to handle the food. However, when you go on a fast, those acids are still there, being produced, even though there isn't any food in your stomach to handle it. Because of this, it is common that you may experience heartburn.

This heartburn can range from just a bit of discomfort to burping all day to even full-on pain. Time is going to help with this side effect. As you spend more time fasting, the body will get better at regulating the acid that is produced, and it will go away. Make sure that you drink plenty of water on your fast, prop yourself up a bit when you go to sleep. And then, when it is time to eat after the fast, don't eat spicy or greasy foods that will make the heartburn worse. If this symptom doesn't go away, then it may be time for you to speak to your doctor about it.

Feeling cold

This side effect is noted less often than others, but some people who go on a fast do find they become colder. This could be because the digestive system slows down during this time because there isn't any food for the stomach to digest. As a result, the body won't release as much heat. Make sure to dress warmly and keep some blankets on hand to ensure that you don't feel too cold during this time.

Headaches

Some people who go on a fast get headaches at the beginning, which can be from a lack of food or lack of energy. Sometimes it can even be from not getting enough water and relaxation. If you feel that these headaches are becoming a big issue, you need to sit back and relax more and make sure that you are drinking plenty of water, as hydration is a major cause of headaches.

Low energy

One common complaint that comes up with people who are ready to start on fasting is that they feel low on energy. It is possible that you will feel a bit lethargic and tired when you first go on a fast, and this can make it hard to have any motivation to get anything done. It can also make it harder to stick with the type of fast that you want and ensure that you get results.

There is a good reason for all of this happening. We brought this up a bit before, but basically, the body is used to relying on glucose, from the carbs and sugars that we consume in our diet, for its fuel source. Glucose is really easy to get hold of in your body, and the cells don't have to do a ton of extra work in order to make these into fuel. It may be easy for the body, but glucose is a very inefficient source of fuel.

In many cases, we don't use it all up. We may still be hungry for more because the glucose will be in the bloodstream and not the stomach, but not used up. This extra glucose is then stored in the body as excess fat and can accumulate all around the body. We end up in a vicious cycle of taking on more and more glucose that we don't need, but which the body wants to use as fuel.

When you go on a fast, especially one that is a bit longer, the body has to learn how to rely on something other than glucose for energy. For the first twelve hours, it will rely on the glucose to keep it healthy and strong. However, if your fast lasts for longer than that, the body has to search for another fuel source. This can take some time for the body to do, and in the meantime, you will feel tired and low on energy.

After some time, the body will become more adjusted to going straight to using fat to keep you energized, and the process is not going to take so long. You may find that you have even more energy than usual when this happens. Until that time, make sure that you stay hydrated, and give yourself some time to rest so that you can stick with the fasting and all of the benefits that come with it!

Overeating

After you go on a fast, you are going to be hungry. All of the protocols will have you going longer than usual without eating anything. Going that long can be healthy for you and will provide you with some of the health benefits that we talked about above, but it will still make you feel hungry when everything is done. Because of this, it is very important that you watch out for what you eat when you are done.

As you get to the end of a long fast, you are going to have a lot of hunger and a lot of cravings that you need to deal with. This is completely normal, but if you are not careful, you will easily end up overeating and making yourself uncomfortable. Think about it, yes, you are hungry, but your stomach has been empty for a long time. If you just dive into everything that you see right when the fast is done, this is going to cause a number of problems.

The first problem that can arise is making yourself feel uncomfortably full. You will have trouble stopping yourself from eating too much because when you eat fast, the stomach can't signal to the brain quick enough that it is done. This can make your stomach hurt and be a general discomfort. In addition, when you eat this fast and this much, it is easy to take in too many calories. Part of the benefits of going on a fast is that it can help you to restrict your calorie intake and ensure that you lose weight. If you overeat, that all goes out the window.

It is natural to be hungry when the fast is done, and you will probably want many things that are comfort foods, with lots of sugars and carbs. The best way to handle the end of your fast and to ensure that you don't overeat is to do a meal plan. Before you go on the fast, consider sitting down and planning out your meals. This allows you to figure out what you will eat after the fast, and before the fast, and you can make smarter choices when the fast is done, and you are hungry.

Brain fog

In the beginning, you may feel as if there is a fog around your brain. Brain fog as well, as a general feeling of being sluggish, is pretty common when you get started on a fast as you get used to it all. The good news is that as you adjust to the fast, and you get a chance to let the body find its new source of fuel outside of the regular and easy to find glucose, then the brain fog is going to go away. In fact, some studies that show that going on a fast and implementing it into your life for a long time can improve how well the brain can function.

While there are a few different types of negative side effects that can happen when you go on a fast, whether it is an intermittent fast or an extended fast, most of these are going to be pretty short term. You won't have to worry about them staying around for a long time, and if you can make it through a week or so with these side effects (for the shorter-term fasts), then you will see some amazing results and the side effects will go away.

How Long Should You Go On a Fast?

The next thing to consider is how long of a fast you would like to go on. This can depend on a number of factors. You have to consider what health condition you are dealing with, your previous diet, whether you want to implement this into your health routine, and more.

First, we are going to take a look at the health condition that you are going to solve with the fast. If you just want to improve your overall health, then it is a good idea to go on one of the protocols from intermittent fasting. You can easily add in this kind of fasting on a regular basis, choosing a daily fast, or going on one that is a bit longer one or two times a week and still get the benefits. However, if you have a major health concern that you need to get fixed quickly, and you want to get a head start on it, doing an extended fast that lasts between seven to ten days may be the best bet.

This can be incredibly effective when it comes to things like high blood pressure. Studies have shown that patients with blood pressure that was considered high were able to reduce their pressure drastically in a seven-day fast. Those who had higher blood pressures were able to see even more dramatic changes. These changes can happen with intermittent fasting, but not as quick. For people who have blood pressure readings that are getting out of control, it may be time to consider going on an extended fast to get it under control.

In addition, you need to worry about the seriousness of the health condition that you already have. For some situations, it may not be a good idea to go on a longer fast. This could make the situation worse. That doesn't mean that one of the shorter fasts offered with intermittent fasting may not be the right option for your needs.

The next thing to consider is the diet that you are on before you start the fast. For those who are on a traditional American diet, it may be hard to switch straight from that over to a ten-day fast. The body is used to having a constant supply of food and glucose available to it, and switching off suddenly can be a big challenge, and can bring out more negative side effects. It may be easier for you to start with a one-day fast a few times a week, or a short daily fast, to help you get started.

This doesn't mean that you can't jump into the longer fast, regardless of what your previous diet was like. However, most people find that going from a lifestyle of excess to one that has nothing at all for that long is difficult. Starting out slowly, and then increasing your times for fasting, can make all the difference in how your health is doing.

What If I Have a Severe Medical Condition?

While fasting can be very beneficial to most people and can provide them with a ton of great health benefits, some medical conditions don't do the best when it comes to this kind of fasting method. Depending on the medical conditions that you have, it may be best to either avoid going on fasting altogether, avoid going on some of the extended fasts or at least go on a fast with the help and supervision of your doctor.

The first condition that you need to watch out for is insulin resistance diabetes. While some symptoms of diabetes can be helped with a fast, especially the shorter-term fasts, you may find that it doesn't work well for you to go on an extended fast without supervision from your doctor. You do not want to go that long without eating when your body relies on the nutrients to keep itself going. If you are going to go on a fast to help with your diabetes, start with a shorter-term fast and see how that goes.

Another group that needs to be careful about going on a fast is those who are dealing with thyroid issues. Your thyroid gland can be in charge of many different hormones in the body. And fasting can cause some issues in the hormone levels as well. In some cases, if the fast isn't monitored properly, and the thyroid issue is bad enough, it could cause more harm than good in these individuals.

Those who are pregnant or may become pregnant soon or who are breastfeeding should never go on one of these fasts. Yes, you may miss a few meals if you are pregnant and dealing with morning sickness. However, there shouldn't be any planned fasting time during any of these periods in your life. Women in these conditions need to provide their body with a constant supply of good nutrition, and this just isn't possible when dealing with fasting in any form.

If you are very concerned about how fasting will affect you and your medical condition, outside of just worrying about being hungry and a little uncomfortable, then it is important to talk to your doctor before you get started with the process of fasting. This allows you to have a chance to discuss the fast with your doctor, ask any questions that you have, and make sure you fully understand the protocol that you are choosing before you get started.

Chapter 6: If Fasting Is Not for You – Ways to Achieve Autophagy Without Fasting

We already know that many great benefits come with entering into the autophagic process. This process allows your body to clean up much of the waste that would otherwise hang around, reduce inflammation, prevent a ton of common diseases and aging issues, and help our bodies feel better. The main way that people are going to induce autophagy is with the help of fasting – as we have talked about in the rest of this guidebook.

However, for some people, fasting is not an option. Maybe they have tried it for some time, and they can't keep up with it, so they need to go with something else. Maybe the fasting plans just aren't best based on their medical history. For others, fasting may work, but they want to try something else along with it to get some more pronounced results.

The good news here is that there are different methods that you can follow to help induce the autophagic process. Whether you do these at the same time as a fast, or on their own, they can induce autophagy and help you get all of the great health benefits. Let's take a look at some of the other methods of inducing autophagy that you may want to consider for your health and lifestyle.

Exercising

The typical American spends a lot of time sitting around the house, or at their jobs, or doing other things during the day. They don't get the amount of movement that they should, and they feel worn out and tired all the time. However, another problem that can come when you don't exercise is that you aren't allowing the body time to clean itself out via the natural processes that come with exercising.

It is possible for exercise to be enough to induce autophagy, especially when you do more intense workouts at least a few times a week. This is because, like exercise, autophagy is going to respond to stress on the body, and exercise is going to work by creating a bit of damage to the tissues and muscles. These damages are small and not such a big deal, but they are a natural part of the detoxification process that comes with autophagy.

The small damage that occurs may be natural, but then the body will go in and make repairs to these small damages. This helps to clean out the body and can ensure that you become leaner and stronger in the process. Even smaller spurts of exercise a few times a week may be enough to turn this process on.

In addition, research shows that exercise is going to help increase the amount of blood flow and vasodilation that occurs throughout the body. This increase in blood flow can make us feel better, and it hurries up the cleaning out process.

One study that was done on mice involved giving the animals substances that made their autophagosomes a glowing green color. These are the structures that are going to surround the wastes of the cells or the other parts that the body is going to recycle. It was found that when the rats ran on the treadmill for at least 30 minutes, the amount of glowing green in the mice ended up increasing.

This speed seemed to keep on increasing until the mice reached about 90 minutes of running. This means that the mice were able to demolish their cells just by running and doing some cardio. Exercise can definitely be a quick way for the body to induce autophagy on its own and make you feel great in a short amount of time.

The good news is that it seems any kind of exercise is going to be efficient. You don't have to spend hours on the treadmill just to see a little bit of autophagy happen. Any kind of training that is a bit higher in intensity, and that can get your heart rate up, will help you with this process. You should aim to get about twenty to 30 minutes of this kind of exercise into your day in order to see the autophagic process happen. Getting a little extra on occasion can help as well.

This means that it is time to implement a good and regular exercise program into your daily routine. There are many great exercises out there, and you may find that implementing a few of them into your schedule, and mixing and matching them a bit, can make it easier to stick with the workout plan and ensure that you don't get bored with the experience. Try to aim for a good mixture of flexible and stretching, weight training, and cardio to get the best results.

The Ketogenic Diet for Autophagy

If you are not interested in going on one of the fasts that we have talked about in this guidebook, but you are still interested in getting into the process of autophagy, then following the ketogenic diet may be the answer you are looking for. This is a great diet plan that reduces the amount of glucose that you take in, whether it comes in the form of carbs or sugars, and forces the body into the same fat burning process that you find when you spend time on a fast. However, you can get into that fat burning mode without having to go long periods without eating.

When we look at the ketogenic diet, we notice that it is a very low carb, moderate protein, and high fat kind of diet. This is very much the opposite of what we are used to seeing in a traditional American diet, which is why it is successful for so many people. The idea with this diet plan is that we want to take in as many of our calories from the fats that are found in food, and as few calories from carbs as we can.

First, let's take a look at the fats. It is recommended that you aim for 60 to 75 percent of your daily calories coming from fats. This is a high number and can take some time to adjust to, but it will do wonders for turning your body into a fat burning machine and can help you to stay full and focused. There are a lot of great sources of healthy fats, such as butter, olive oil, and even fats that are found on various meat sources.

Next comes the protein sources. You will want to get about twenty percent of your daily calories from protein. This ensures that you are getting enough protein to keep the muscles strong and lean, especially if you are adding in a workout plan to all of this, but also ensure that the majority of your calories are going to come from the fat we talked about before. There are many great sources of protein that you can go with. You can focus primarily on protein sources that have some heavier amounts of fats as well, but any protein source can work well. Just make sure that you stay away from breaded and fried options because these are going to add in more carbs as compared to what we are allowed on this diet plan.

And finally, we need to focus on keeping our carb content as low as possible. It is recommended that you only keep about five percent of your daily calories set aside for your carb intake. This can sometimes be hard to do, but it ensures that you can enter the process of ketosis. When you are picking out your carbs, don't waste them on things like pasta, desserts, and other baked goods, etc. Instead, make sure that you are getting a wide variety of vegetables, and maybe some fruit, so you can get more nutrition out of the few carbs that you get.

The whole point of limiting the carbs so much on the ketogenic diet is to ensure that your body enters ketosis. With this process, the body can give up its dependence on glucose, and will instead focus on using fats, either the fats that we eat or the fats that are stored in the body, to help keep it energized and doing well. This is a great way to clean out the body and can make the individual feel healthier because they don't have to rely on the glucose any longer.

Some people who are dealing with many different health problems, or those who want to lose weight, may find that it is best for them to go on a combination of a fast and the ketogenic diet. Adding these both together can help the body achieve the autophagic process. With that said, fasting isn't the right option for some people. If this is the case with you, then it may be a good idea to go with the ketogenic diet and see what benefits it can provide your body.

Getting Enough Sleep

Failure to get enough sleep can interfere with the process of autophagy. This is because much of this process is going to occur while we are asleep when we don't have our resources put towards other things.

In one animal study, it was confirmed that sleep deprivation altered the process of autophagy, allowing all of those dead and damaged cells to hang around the body. What this means is that you must make sure that you get enough sleep each night, and ensure that you stay on the same sleeping schedule to see the best results.

In our modern world, it is sometimes hard to get the amount of sleep that we really need as we spend so much time working, going to school, running to activities, trying to meet up with friends, cleaning the house, and trying to get a million other things done during the day. Then, at the end of the day, we are either still doing more work, or get distracted by social media and other things. It isn't uncommon to go many nights without getting the full eight to nine hours of sleep that you need to see the autophagic process in action.

There are a number of things that you can do to ensure you get enough sleep on a day-to-day basis. Some tips include:

• Set a bedtime: And stick with it, even on the weekend and other days off. The closer you can maintain your set bedtime, the better off you will be. It ensures that you can fall asleep at the same time each night, and can make it easier to wake up the next morning. Even if you have a day off or nowhere to be the next day, it is important to stick with the same bed and wake up time.

• Get into a routine: The best thing that you can do when you are trying to get more sleep is to set up a bedtime routine. The point of this is that once the body gets used to the routine, as soon as you get started with the first task, the brain will start gearing up to fall asleep and you won't have to put in as much work as before. The bedtime routine doesn't need to be something that is overly complicated and hard to follow. You could make it as simple as taking a bath, brushing your hair, brushing your teeth, reading a chapter in a book, and then going to bed.

• Turn off your phone and avoid screen time: Screen time can really mess with your sleeping patterns. It is best to turn off your phone, shut down your computer or laptop, and stop watching a movie at least a bit before you are ready to go to bed. This can be so beneficial to the brain and the body and makes falling asleep much easier.

• Spend some time reading: After a long day of work or school or anything else that has gone on, it is often hard to calm right down. You should have a transitory time between all that craziness of the day and the time you go to bed. Spending a few minutes, even just fifteen minutes, reading at the end of the day can help keep you calm and make it easier to fall asleep.

• Turn the lights off: Don't go to bed with the light on. This light can interrupt your sleep and confuse the body. If you must have a light, keep a small nightlight somewhere out of the way.

• Don't turn the television on in your room: One of the worst things that you can do when it comes to your sleeping schedule and how deeply you fall asleep is having a television in your room. Some people swear that this is the only way that they fall asleep, but in reality, it is messing with their REM cycle. Take the television out of your room and replace it with some soothing music instead and see what a difference it makes.

• Keep the room a bit cooler than normal: Most people sleep the best when they have the room at a slightly cooler temperature. You don't have to keep it freezing, but try not to keep it too warm either. You can always cuddle up with an extra blanket to help if needed.

• Get comfortable: It is harder to get to sleep if you find that you feel uncomfortable. Bring in enough pillows, or invest in some new ones, find some sleeping clothes that make you feel good, and bring in blankets. Each person is going to find comfort differently when it comes to their sleeping arrangements, so do what works best for you.

• Silence is best but use nature sounds or classical music if necessary: Silence is often the best way to fall asleep, so you don't feel overwhelmed by the noises that are going on around you. However, for some people, the silence is too hard to fall asleep to. If this is the case for you, then it is fine to turn on some quiet music. Classical music or sounds of nature are the best to lull you to sleep.

Nothing is better than getting enough sleep. It can be hard to see this happen and maintain. However, if you really want to see the results of your efforts, especially if you are working on one of the other options, then make sure you implement a good sleeping schedule into your routine.

Eating the Right Foods

We discussed this a bit when we talked about fasting and going on a ketogenic diet in order to help induce autophagy, but eating a healthy diet is one of the best things that you can do to bring autophagy on in your body. If the body doesn't receive the nutrients it needs to stay healthy, it won't be able to carry out all of the important processes that are needed to keep you going, whether these processes include autophagy or not.

Some of the foods that you should consider adding into your diet to assist with the autophagic process include:

- Turmeric
- Coconut oil
- Green tea
- Coffee
- Ginger

Of course, eating a diet that is well balanced, one that includes many healthy nutrients and minerals, such as what you can get from plenty of fruits and vegetables, is the best way to enter this process. These nutrients are key when it comes time to help the body eliminate waste most effectively.

Protein Fast

This is another type of fasting but is a bit different than the others. You are still allowed to eat, but you will limit the amount of protein that you consume for a short amount of time. You will find that it is possible to get the same benefits that come from autophagy simply by going on a protein fast. For this to work, you will occasionally go on a fast where you eat normally, but you take in 25 fewer grams for the day.

The main idea that comes with this kind of fast is that it allows your body to have a full day to go through and recycle old proteins. These older proteins may not have had a chance to clear themselves out of the body – since they linger around and cause inflammation in the body.

This kind of eating plan will allow the body to clean out all of the cells, without having to worry about muscle loss along the way, helping you to stay lean and fit. These fasts, or lack of protein periods, will only be for a few days so you won't miss out on the protein the body needs too much.

According to one study that has been done on the protein fast, when you can limit the amount of protein that you take in, this will force the body to go through and consume the proteins that are already present in the body – the ones that haven't been used up yet and are becoming toxic in the cells. The way that this eating plan clears out the cells is that it binds the toxins that are found in the cytoplasm of the cell and then moves them out.

Other studies show how being a bit deficient in protein can help to induce the process of autophagy because it is going to work in a manner that is similar to going on a fast, but you won't cut out all of the other nutrients, or go long periods without eating. This is because being deficient in protein reduces both the mTOR and insulin levels, both of which work together to control cell growth and metabolism.

When you can reduce your mTOR levels, and then work to build them back up, it does wonders for helping the body build and repair cells, leading to more lean muscle throughout. This kind of process is also going to help out with controlling aging, as well as preventing disease like diabetes, cancer, and heart disease.

One thing to note is that you don't need to limit the amount of protein that you eat on a daily basis. In fact, having this kind of deficit all the time is going to be a bad thing. You need to have protein in your diet to help build up muscles and to help with many other important processes that occur throughout the body. However, doing this kind of fast on an occasional basis can give the body time to clean up the excess proteins that are found in the cells, allowing it to be more efficient at doing its job.

If you want to go with a protein fast, you will do one that lasts about 24 to 36 hours, just once a week. Some people decide to go with this two times a week and follow the protocol similar to what is found in the 5:2 diet. Remember, you are allowed to eat during a protein fast; you just cut down the grams of protein that you get during that time. The other nutrients can stay about the same.

The protein fast can be a great option to go on to help you enter into autophagy. It promotes a lot of the same benefits and induces autophagy similarly to some of the fasts that we have discussed in this guidebook, without having to spend much time on a long fast and feeling hungry along the way. You may want to give this method a try before starting on a regular fast if you are interested in seeing the benefits of autophagy but have a medical condition that makes it hard to go on a traditional fast.

As you can see, there are several different methods that you can use to induce autophagy. While fasting is often the best and more efficient method and the one that most people will choose to go with first, other methods can prove effective as well. If you are worried about going on a traditional fast, or you are looking for another method that doesn't require you to go hungry, then considering a protein fast, the ketogenic diet, or exercising.

Chapter 7: The Results

If you are looking to get on a fasting regimen or any other diet plan, one of the first things that you need to establish, after determining the rules that go behind it, is the results that you want to achieve. No one wants to spend weeks on a plan, going through times of not eating and working on their willpower only to find out that the real results of that fasting are only two pounds lost over three months.

Often, one of the key parts to find the right motivation you need to stick with a lifestyle change or a diet is having the knowledge and the confidence that it will work. Reading about the success of others when they went on a fast or any other kind of diet and nutrition plan can help you convince yourself that it is possible. You may feel more confident that since they lost the weight, you can as well.

In this chapter, we are going to take a look at some of the various success stories that have shown up concerning fasting – and we've divided them up based on the different protocols that they used to get the results. This helps you to see that fasting really is effective and may be the perfect option for you. It may also help you to choose which of the fasting protocols you like the best if you are stuck on which one to go with.

Linda Christie's Story

Linda Christie was 65 and living in Ashford, Kent when she decided to try out the 5:2 protocol for fasting. In just six months, she lost a total of three stone and dropped from a size sixteen to a size ten. According to Linda, when you get to the age of 60, your health becomes more of a priority. She had the goal of being fit and active for years to come so that she could keep up with her young grandsons, rather than living life as an ailing old lady.

In 2012, she had seen someone talking about intermittent fasting on television. She was intrigued by the promises of health and longevity, and so she decided to give it a try. Before that time, she had weighted about twelve stone and was 5'7". She wasn't what was considered overweight by a lot, but she did know that the extra pounds were impacting her health – she noticed that the weight was painful on her knees, and bending to put her shoes on was a big challenge.

Linda found that the first few days on the 5:2 fast were difficult as she struggled to make it through the fasting days. However, soon she noticed that she was losing around two pounds each week, and that gave her more motivation to carry on. Since she looked after her grandsons a few days a week, she planned her fasting days on the ones when she wasn't looking after them.

For her protocol, she would skip breakfast on these fasting days, then have a bowl of soup for lunch, and then another bowl in the evening with some more vegetables thrown in. Depending on how she felt, she sometimes decided to do a third fast day on Saturday. However, Sunday was always her cheat day of having some donuts at church and maybe a treat at choir rehearsals that evening.

Now that she has reached her goal of getting down to nine stone and four pounds, Linda made some adjustments to her fast and just went on the fast on Tuesdays. That is one of the nice parts of doing this kind of fast. You can make the adjustments that are needed to your daily life, either before or after you reach your goals, to ensure that you maintain it for the long term.

Terri Durrant's Story

Terri Durrant was 56 when she started out with the 5:2 diet. Over the time she tried out this diet plan, she lost about two stone and was able to improve her health. According to Terri, before she went on this diet plan, she was suffering from many different health problems. As a younger woman, she had been a swimmer for Great Britain, but all of that exercise had taken a toll on her body, and as a result, she was suffering from knee and back problems.

At the age of 40, Terri noticed that her weight went up to nearly fourteen stone, and she ended up having to go in and get her knee fully replaced. This meant that Terri was out of action for a long time, which made it very difficult to lose weight, despite trying a few other diet plans. After suffering even more health problems, Terri started out 2014 feeling unhealthy and unfit.

A friend of hers recommended the 5:2 version of fasting, and she decided to go for it, with Tuesdays and Thursdays being her fasting days. Slowly and steadily, the weight started to come off. It took her three months to lose half a stone, but by the time she was on it for six months, she had lost more than a stone. She was able to reduce her clothes size from a sixteen to eighteen down to a twelve to fourteen.

Of course, Terri states that the best part of this fast is that it had such a big impact on her health. She can now keep up with her eight dogs, all of whom are show dogs, and since she is a swim teacher, she has noticed that she is now less likely to catch all the bugs that are going around, including chest problems and bronchitis.

Terri has decided to stick with the two fast days a week for now because she wants to be able to get to the nine stone mark. However, during those fasts, she usually keeps herself to two small meals, one at two pm, and then another when she gets home from work around nine pm. Then, she makes sure that she drinks a ton of water all day. She finds that sticking to a set routine helps her to stay focused and get the best results.

Mimi from Food Can Weight

Mimi is another inspirational story about how well fasting can work to help you lose weight and get in the best health of your life. She found herself at almost 240 pounds by June of 2014 and knew it was time to make some changes to the unhealthy eating patterns that she had developed over the years. She had tried many different diet plans throughout her life and even worked with natural appetite suppressants in the hopes of helping her control her appetite that never seemed to go away. She was even at a point of being scared to lose weight because she feared that losing weight, in the beginning, would only result in her weighing more in the end.

Mimi decided to go through the process slightly differently and focused more on fasting like the Warrior diet. After meeting with some friends who practiced Ramadan, she became curious about the spiritual and health benefits that could come from this. She decided that it might be time to try this out and see how it worked.

She decided to go on a 30-day fast. She was not allowed to have anything during the day except coffee, water, and other beverages without calories in them. Then, at night time before bed, she could eat whatever she wanted. This allowed her to still get in many of the nutrients that her body needed, permitting for a little bit of a splurge, and ensured that she was going to get a lot of fat burning done throughout the day.

By 2016, Mimi had been able to lose 73 pounds in total, bringing her down to just 164 pounds from the almost 240 that she had started at. She noticed that her health felt better, she had a lot more energy, and that this kind of fasting was not as hard to maintain as she had thought. She decided to keep going with this kind of fasting to see how far it could take her.

Zach and the Bulletproof Diet

Zach, a busy business executive, decided to go on the rules of an intermittent fast, but he made it a little bit different. Instead of getting rid of all the calories that were in his diet during the fasting window, he decided to use the bulletproof intermittent fasting method. With this method, a bit of bulletproof coffee in the morning was allowed.

Bulletproof intermittent fasting is very similar to what we see with intermittent fasting, but with the addition of a cup of bulletproof coffee in the morning, rather than eating nothing. The healthy fats that come from the grass-fed butter, along with the Brain Octane Oil, will help you get a good and steady current of energy that will do well for sustaining you through the day. The lower toxins that are found in the beans will help to optimize brain function and the fat loss with high octane caffeine. And the oil will ensure that your metabolism will speed up by twelve percent and increase your ketone production more than ever before.

Of course, if you go on this method, you must make sure that you still eat a healthy diet along the way. The bulletproof coffee can help to keep you full, provides you with energy, and ensures that you are less likely to overeat through the day. However, it is not going to save you if you choose to eat Oreos and Pop Tarts for the rest of the day.

Zach was used to depending on sugar to provide him with the energy needed to get stuff done, and as a result, this resulted in a vicious cycle of him being overweight and miserable. After going on this kind of diet plan, he was able to lose a pound a day for 75 days, without feeling overly hungry all the time.

In addition to losing a lot of fat, Zach noticed that he felt more focused throughout the day, was more alert, and never felt deprived, even though he wasn't eating much. He didn't have to do steroids or other protocols to see the results. He simply had to stop eating at about eight at night, and then, instead of having breakfast, he would have some bulletproof coffee, then wait until lunch to have a meal.

These are just a few of the different success stories that have been found when it comes to intermittent fasting. There are thousands of other stories out there. By going on one of these fasts, or even a longer-term fast, you are getting yourself in the best health possible and ensuring that the process of autophagy occurs for you.

Chapter 8: FAQ About Autophagy and Fasting

As we have discussed, autophagy is the process where the body breaks down old and damaged cells and then removes them. When autophagy is allowed to happen, the cells can use these wastes to stay energized and as fuel to get things done. This is a natural process that should be occurring in our bodies, but thanks to poor eating and diet habits, this process is often delayed or never happens at all.

These broken and damaged parts are completely normal. When you breathe, workout, just live life, and more, the body is going to break down cells and other parts. That is just healthy functioning of your body, which makes room for new parts. The new parts can then do their job, and you feel great with the actions you have to do from one day to the next.

The problem comes when you don't see autophagy occur. Thanks to the unhealthy diets that we have put ourselves on and all of the other toxic environments around us, such as lack of exercise, bad habits, and generally not taking care of ourselves, we have effectively turned off the process of autophagy. Remember, the body needs to go through some kind of stress, such as fast or exercising, in order to enter into this autophagic process. If it never experiences that stress, then it will just keep being turned off and is going to wreak havoc on your body.

With the autophagic process turned off, there is still the issue of broken and damaged proteins and cell parts that are hanging around. These are always going to occur. Even someone who is considered extremely healthy is going to have these wastes produced in the body. It is the way that the body works to repair itself and the way that you get new parts to keep you feeling good and everything working the way that it should.

With a healthy body that promotes autophagy, those wastes are going to be used as fuel and then will pass on through the body. However, when autophagy doesn't occur because the body never goes through one of those good stressors, then the wastes are just going to hang out around the body, and this is never a good thing.

When all of these wastes are left in the body with nowhere to go, it leads to a bunch of problems. First, without a process to go through and clean them up and even to break them down, these wastes are just going to keep hanging out where they were originally put. This prevents new cells and proteins from coming in and doing the job more efficiently for you.

Think of it like having a car. You may look inside and see that some parts are brand-new and some have been on since the car was first made. Just by looking at it, you already know which parts are going to work the best and which ones will struggle. The newer parts will function the most efficiently and will get the job done without any problems. However, the older parts are going to cause problems, can wear on the newer parts, which have to take up some extra work to keep things going, and it won't be long until they break completely.

Simply by replacing these older parts, you can improve the functioning of the car.

The same is true in your body. You need to be able to get rid of all the wastes, so they don't get in the way of the newer parts, and they can even make other parts of the body work harder than usual, causing other parts to get old and worn out at the same time.

In addition, all of these wastes hanging around are known to cause inflammation. This alone can be the root cause of many serious diseases, from high blood pressure to cancer to arthritis, and even more. Autophagy can help solve this issue.

This guidebook has explained many of the methods that you can use to help bring about this autophagic process and to help you get the most out of it once you start. In addition, here are some more things that you need to know before you decide to get started with fasting and to induce the autophagic process.

Do I Really Need Autophagy to Occur?

It is very important that you promote autophagy through the cells. A natural process of the body is to burn out various pieces. These pieces will get old and damaged, just from normal wear and tear from what you do on a daily basis. Autophagy ensures that all of these parts are taken out of the body, without them getting in the way.

Without autophagy, those broken and damaged parts are just going to stick around the body. They will get in the way of new parts forming. The body will continue to use the same old and damaged parts, which is never a good thing for helping you to fight off illness or feel your best. Over time, these broken parts are going to start to cause inflammation and may be the reason that you are suffering from a variety of different diseases, including those related to aging.

Autophagy ensures that this doesn't happen. When older parts are allowed to be removed from the body, it provides newer parts the opportunity to grow and thrive. This helps to give you more energy, makes it easier to lose weight and can prevent a bunch of serious health conditions.

Isn't Fasting Bad for Me?

Many people worry that going on a fast is bad for them. They worry that they are going to harm their bodies and enter into starvation mode. However, it takes a lot more than just a few hours of fasting before you will enter into starvation mode, and it is not going to happen on any of the fasting methods that we talked about in this guidebook – unless you do really bad at following the protocol.

To get into starvation mode, the body has to go a very long time without eating or go a very long time with minimal nutrition. The body has to feel that it is missing out on food and that it needs to preserve what is already has, so it slows down the metabolism. However, if you are going on a fast that is only 24 hours long or less, and you make sure to eat plenty of healthy and nutritious foods during your eating window, then starvation mode is not going to be an issue.

The truth is that fasting has tons of great health benefits that can make you look and feel amazing. Fasting will help you lose weight, get rid of belly fat, lower blood pressure, lower high cholesterol levels, reduce brain fog and other brain problems, and so much more. Even just a short fast on occasion will help you to see great improvements in your overall health, all thanks to the autophagic process.

How Can Fasting Help with Autophagy?

Fasting is one of the best ways to enter into the process of autophagy. Study after study has shown that when the body gets away from using the readily available glucose for energy, it will use the stored fat to keep you going. This process will also instigate the autophagy, which helps to clear out all the toxins and dead and damaged parts of the body that are just getting in the way and causing lots of disease and other issues.

It is best if you can go on a fast that lasts for about sixteen hours. Remember, it takes about twelve hours from your last meal before the fat burning process begins. The sixteen hours ensures that you can spend at least a few hours burning fat, and seeing autophagy occur throughout the body. The longer the fast, the more fat-burning you will see, and the better results you will get.

Can I Enter Autophagy Without Going on a Fast?

Fasting is one of the fastest and most efficient ways to enter into the autophagic process. You only have to go on the fast for a very short amount of time to see this process start up. With that said, there are other options that you can use to help bring about the process of autophagy and help your body get in the best shape possible.

If you are not interested in going on a fast, if you shouldn't go on a fast, or if you are interested in enhancing your fast, then there are a few options available to you. Other ways that you can make sure that you get the most out of the autophagic process include starting the ketogenic diet, eating the right kinds of foods, getting enough sleep, and adding a good exercise routine into your day.

Is There Anyone Who Shouldn't Go on a Fast?

Fasting can be effective for almost anyone who wants to induce the autophagic process and those who want to lose weight and help out a host of other health conditions. However, there are a few people who may find that fasting is not the best option for them.

First, if you are pregnant, breastfeeding, or thinking about getting pregnant in the near future, then fasting is not a good idea. Fasting restricts the nutrients that you take in during the day. While you should be able to make those up during your eating window, you will find that these conditions require you to get a constant stream of nutrition throughout the day. It is better to stay off a fast and wait until after your baby is born, or after you are done breastfeeding.

There are also a number of health concerns that can be aggravated when it comes to fasting. Type 1 diabetes is not always the best for going on one of these fasts, and you may notice that those who have a thyroid condition will often be told not to go on a fast. If you are concerned about how your medical condition will be affected if you decide to go on a fast, make sure to bring up the issue with your doctor.

What Is the Best Length of Fasting for Me?

As we discussed in this guidebook, there are many different fasting protocols that you can choose to go on to help improve your health. As long as you go on a fast for at least twelve hours, although sixteen is usually preferred, you will enter into the autophagic process. Hence, any of the different protocols that we have talked about in this guidebook can work to help you see results.

The protocol that works the best for you may be different compared to what works the best for someone else. If you are hesitant about starting a fast, or worried about how it may aggravate a condition that you already have, then you may want to choose one of the easier daily fasts, such as the 16/8 protocol. On the other hand, if you really want to lose a lot of weight quickly and see your results in next to no time, or you want to help heal a medical condition that has been plaguing you, then going on an alternate day fast or something similar may be a good idea.

Chapter 9: Tips and Tricks to Make Fasting Easier

While there are other methods that you can use to enter the process of autophagy, most people find that going on a fast is the easiest and most efficient method out there. It provides you with quick results, you get many different options to help you out, and it isn't too difficult to follow. With that said, it is a big shift from the way that you ate in the past –and this can be hard for some people to get used to in the beginning.

Fasting is not meant to be a difficult process – it just requires a bit of adjusting and a few tricks to make it work. Some of the best tricks that you can follow to see results when you get started on fasting include:

Start After Dinner

One trick that you may want to try out when you are ready to start with fasting is to make sure that the fast starts after you finish dinner. There are a number of benefits to choosing this as the starting point.

The first benefit is that you won't go to bed hungry. Going to bed hungry is never a positive experience and is one of the main reasons that many people end up failing – or at least really struggling – when it comes to going on a fast. They may have all the ambition to do well, but when they go to bed with their stomachs growling and not being allowed to eat because of the protocol they chose and the amount of time left in their fasting window, they feel miserable.

When you finish the fast after supper, you get the benefit of at least going to bed with a full stomach, and that alone can make the process of fasting so much easier to handle. You will be hungry at some point the next day, but at least you have slept well the night before.

With this method, you will have to skip breakfast the next day. However, the hunger from this can fade pretty quickly. And if you keep yourself busy at work or cleaning the house or getting the kids off to school, etc., you will find that it doesn't take long until you get to lunchtime and you can eat again. This is one of the easiest and most comfortable methods to use to go on a fast, and you will get the best results out of it.

Make Sure That You Drink Plenty of Water

When you go on a fast, or anytime in your life, you should make sure that you drink plenty of water. Water is important for many aspects of your life. It can help you feel hydrated and will keep a bunch of nasty side effects at bay in your body. It can help promote the process of autophagy and makes it easier to dispose of all the waste that is caught up in that process. And water can help to keep your hunger at bay when you are dealing with a fast.

It is very important that you drink a lot of water during your fast. It is easy to become dehydrated during this time, and once you do, many of the negative side effects that we talked about earlier in this guidebook will start to plague you. If you want to limit or reduce these negative side effects, then it is important that you keep a water bottle near you to help keep yourself hydrated.

Make sure that you drink a little bit of extra water than you normally would during the fasting time. Remember, you are not getting your water from food sources during this time, which can mean you are missing up to twenty percent of your liquid content when you are on the fast. Adding in a bit more water to your routine while you do this can really help to keep the dehydration away.

Consider Drinking Some Sparkling Water

This one goes along with the drinking water idea above, but there is a slightly different reason. Yes, it will help to keep you hydrated, and it can be a nice change if you have just been drinking regular water while fasting. For people who are on an extended water fast, plain water is going to get boring pretty quickly, but adding flavoring to the water to make it more interesting will probably throw you off the fast.

However, with sparkling water, you can get a bit of a change to the type of water that you are consuming. That alone can make you feel better and can keep you on the fast for a little bit longer. But another benefit that comes from drinking sparkling water is that it can help keep you full. The bubbles are great for filling up the stomach and making you feel the hunger pains less than before. For those who are going on a longer fast, this can be just the trick you need to make it more manageable to handle.

Coffee Can Help Keep the Hunger Away

Another thing to consider when you need help curbing your appetite is to make sure that you drink a bit of coffee. You don't want to go overboard with this because, for some people, caffeine can cause the jitters and an ill feeling, especially if consumed on an empty stomach. However, having a cup of coffee in the morning while still on your fast can be a great way not only to wake you up but also make some of those hunger cues go away.

If you are going to use coffee to help keep the hunger pains away, make sure that it is black coffee. You can't add sugar and cream or any other additions to the coffee while you are fasting. This may be the way that you liked to drink coffee in the past, but these things are not allowed when you are fasting, and they are going to kick you right out of your fat burning mode. Plus, adding those two things can increase your cravings for the rest of the day if you are not careful.

Find Ways to Distract Yourself

The hardest part of a fast comes when you let yourself sit around and think about food, or think about how long you have until your eating window starts. When you get bored, this will be the only thing you want to think about, and then the cravings and the temptation and the extra hungry stomach will start to take over, and you will feel miserable. When all three of these things start to gang up on you, it is just a matter of time before you cave and go off your fasting protocol.

Instead of letting this happen, make sure that you get out of the house, or at least find other ways to distract yourself. The more that you can concentrate on getting something else done, the less time and energy you have to focus on the fact that you haven't eaten in a bit.

There are many different ways that you can work to distract yourself from hunger pains. Consider making your fasting days the ones that you work most on. You can then sit and work diligently on all projects and other tasks that you need to get done, without worrying about when it is time to eat. In fact, many people claim that they are more focused and more productive when they are on a fast, so this can help you to really speed through the work and get a lot done.

If one of your fasting days happens to occur over a weekend or another day when you aren't at work, then it may be best to consider finding other ways to distract yourself. This can be especially important for some of those longer-term fasts as well. Cleaning the house, working on that one big project that needs to get done, reading, going on a walk, and more can really help you to focus on something other than your hungry stomach.

Finish Your Work in the Morning Before the Fast Is Over, and You Can Eat

Exercise is a very important part of fasting and making sure that you get the results that you want. It can help you burn through the glucose faster, so your body starts to rely on fat burning more. It helps you to feel better and tone the body. It can help you to keep your muscle tone going. And all the benefits of fasting can be magnified when you add in the exercise.

One method that has been pretty successful with exercising and fasting is to get the workout in right at the end of the fast. During this time, you have depleted the extra glucose that has been hanging around the body, and you have, hopefully, been in fat-burning mode for at least a few hours. When you enter into a workout, the body is going to still rely on the fat, intensifying the fat burning results that you can get.

Then, when the workout is done, you can help replenish the body by breaking your fast and having something to eat. This ensures that you get some extra fat burning results while still providing the body with the nutrients it needs after a hard workout. Just make sure that you plan out the meal a bit to avoid overeating on the things you crave, and to help you give your body the nutrients it needs.

Of course, working out at any time of day is very beneficial, so if you find that waiting until the end of the fast is too hard, or you just don't have the time during that period of the day, then it isn't such a big deal. Some people like to work out during their eating window, so they have the nutrients to keep them going on a more intense workout. Some people like to go right at the start of the fast to help push them into fat burning faster. Pick the workout schedule that works the best for you.

Don't Let Others Know That You Are Fasting

It is often best to not let others know that you are on a fast. First off, this gives many negative impressions, and many people may worry that you are doing something to harm yourself. They may not understand why you are doing this, and many may think it is foolish and will try to talk you out of it – but you have personal reasons for going on this fast, and holding on tight to those will make the whole process much easier to deal with.

Telling others that you are going on a fast can be misconstrued as "showing off" and can sometimes set you up for failure. Don't look towards others for the motivation that you need to succeed; instead, look inward and see if you can find your own motivation. What is the main reason why you want to go through all of this? What are you hoping to get out of the process? If you can answer these questions, then you are ready to get started.

Get Out of the House and Away from the Food

Nothing makes fasting harder than just sitting around the house, waiting for your fasting window to be over and your eating window to begin. You are not only going to be bored when you do this, but you are also in close proximity to food during this time. And it is likely that you are going to keep thinking about that food until you get some. How long do you think your endurance and willpower will be able to hold out as you get hungrier and hungrier during the day?

It is fine to stay around the house as long as you have something to do during that time. If you have a big project to work on, some business work to complete, or you even plan to spend the day cleaning, then that is fine. However, if you find that you are just sitting on the sofa watching television, or wandering around aimlessly, hoping that you find some way to bust the boredom and not give in to the hunger or cravings, then this is a recipe for disaster.

When the latter starts to happen, it is time to get out of the house. Even if you just go on a walk for a bit, it is better than being bored in the house where you are likely to make poor decisions and eat foods that you shouldn't. Find some errands to run, meet up with a friend, or head to the library and check out some books – anything that helps you not to sit around and be tempted by food!

Have Some Splurges on Occasion

No one wants to feel like they are deprived all the time. Yes, to see the autophagic process and to lose weight, there are going to be some sacrifices along the way. However, if you are never allowed to splurge and have some fun, then you are going to get bored, and even angry, at your fasting regimen. It is perfectly fine to have a splurge on occasion. It is fine to go out with some friends and push your eating window back a bit. It is fine to eat a few too many calories occasionally. While you should try to keep these down to a minimum, they are not the end of the world.

Don't Feel Bad If You Mess Up Sometimes

As with any kind of diet and eating plan, there are times when you will make mistakes and run into trouble. Maybe you were doing really well on the fast and then, all of a sudden, you ran into trouble and gave in and ate breakfast too soon. This can be disheartening, but again, is not the end of the world.

So what if you didn't make it completely through the fast. You tried hard, and if you followed the protocol well the night before, you still went on a fast for a good amount of time, and you will still get all of the benefits that come with it. Just make sure to plan the rest of your day accordingly. Beating yourself up about this is just going to make the situation worse, and will make it more likely that you will give up and never see any results.

Fasting is one of the best ways to encourage the autophagic process, and it can provide you with a bunch of benefits in the process. However, sometimes, it is hard to make such big adjustments to the way that we eat in order to see these benefits. Following some of the tips that are found in this chapter can make the process much easier to handle overall.

Conclusion

Thank you for making it through to the end of *Autophagy: Unlock the Secrets of Weight Loss, Anti-Aging, and Healing with Intermittent and Extended Water Fasting.*

This guidebook should have been informative and provided you with all of the tools you need to achieve your goals – whatever they may be.

The next step is to take some time to determine which method of inducing autophagy is right for you.

Finally, if you found this book useful in any way, a review on Amazon is always appreciated!

If you enjoyed this individual book on Autophagy, a review on Amazon would be greatly appreciated because it helps me to create more books that people want.

Thanks for your support!

Here's another book by Elizabeth Moore that you might be interested in:

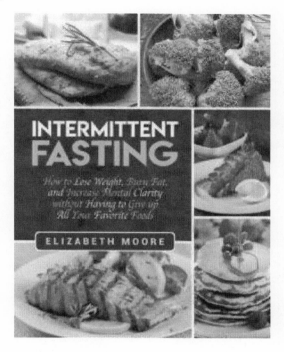